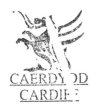

A Woman of Firsts

Edna Adan Ismail was Foreign Minister of Somaliland from 2003 to 2006, and had previously served as Somaliland's Minister of Family Welfare and Social Development.

She is the director and founder of the Edna Adan Maternity Hospital in Hargeisa, which opened in 2002, and an activist and pioneer in the struggle for the abolition of female genital mutilation. She is also President of the Somaliland Association for Victims of Torture.

In 2010, she opened the Edna Adan Ismail University in Hargeisa, Somaliland. She was married to Mohamed Haji Ibrahim Egal who was Head of Government in British Somaliland five days prior to Italian Somalia's independence and later the Prime Minister of Somalia (1967–69) and President of Somaliland from 1993 to 2002.

A Woman of Firsts

The midwife who built a hospital
and changed the world

Edna Adan Ismail

with Wendy Holden
with assistance from Lee Cassanelli

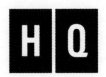

ONE PLACE. MANY STORIES

HQ
An imprint of HarperCollins*Publishers* Ltd
1 London Bridge Street
London SE1 9GF

This edition 2019

1

First published in Great Britain by
HQ, an imprint of HarperCollins*Publishers* Ltd 2019

Copyright © Edna Adan Ismail 2019

Edna Adan Ismail asserts the moral right to be
identified as the author of this work.
A catalogue record for this book is
available from the British Library.

ISBN: 978-0-00-830534-5
ISBN: 978-0-00-830535-2

MIX
Paper from
responsible sources
FSC™ C007454

This book is produced from independently certified FSC™ paper
to ensure responsible forest management.

For more information visit: www.harpercollins.co.uk/green

This book is set in 11.9/16 pt. Bembo

Printed and bound in Great Britain by
CPI Group (UK) Ltd, Croydon, CR0 4YY

This book is dedicated to my father Adan Ismail and to all those, like him, who devote their lives to caring for others with humanity, compassion and kindness.

This memoir is based on my recollection of events which may not be as others recall them. Where conversations cannot be remembered precisely, I have re-created them to the best of my ability. Any mistakes are my own.

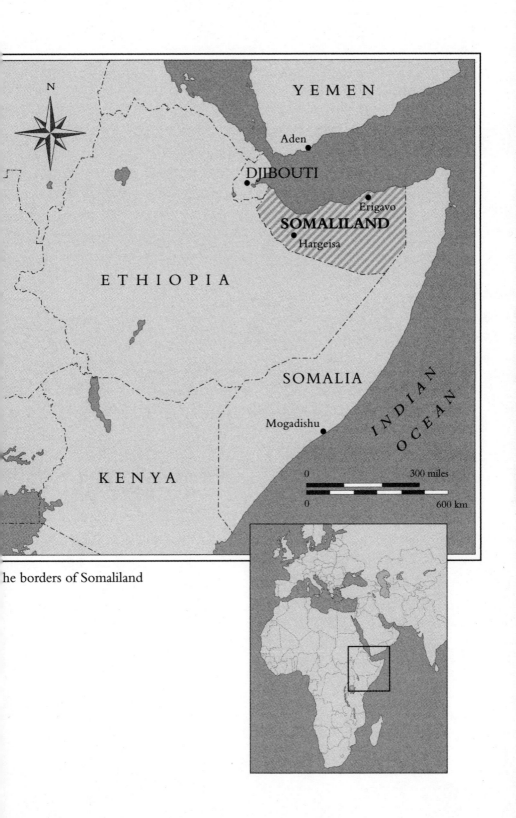

The borders of Somaliland

Prologue

Mogadishu, Somalia, 1975

'Come with me,' I told the military director of Medina Hospital, seconds after bursting into his office unannounced. 'I need you to shoot a baby.'

The colonel, sitting at his desk in uniform with gold braid and pips on his epaulettes, looked up at me aghast. 'What?'

Spotting a weapon lying on his desk, I grabbed it and waved it at him. 'Is this your pistol? I presume it's loaded?'

'Y-yes, Edna,' he faltered, as his lieutenant drew his own gun and stepped forward protectively. 'B–but…'

'Then bring it with you, follow me back to the maternity ward, and shoot a premature baby,' I repeated. 'Isn't that what you carry a gun for – to kill people?'

'I don't understand,' he pleaded, palms turned to the ceiling.

Leaning across his desk and staring straight into his eyes, I told him, 'Then let me explain. I haven't slept for the last three days. I've been caring for a premature baby in the only incubator I possess, a generous gift from a patient. I've been feeding this tiny infant through a pipette. She's a fighter and she's trying to stay alive but the oxygen level on the incubator is running out. I sent a nurse to you twice this morning to ask for a replacement cylinder. Half an hour ago it was returned unfilled with the message that we're using too much oxygen and putting your hospital in the red.'

I paused to watch him squirming in his seat. 'When the oxygen runs out in less than an hour,' I continued, 'that little baby weighing less than a kilo will gasp painfully for her final breath as I watch helplessly with her mother. If you're really planning to murder this baby then I must insist you come with me now and end it quickly. Then you can show the whole world how brave you really are.'

The colonel's face froze. He didn't move or speak. Seething, I grabbed the document he'd been reading, flipped it over and scribbled on the back the following promise: 'If I don't receive oxygen within the next fifteen minutes and – without question – every time that I ask for it thereafter, I, Edna Adan Ismail, herewith declare that I will take no more responsibility for the patients in my care at this hospital.' I signed and dated my declaration and, before anyone could stop me, I picked up a bottle of Superglue, squirted it generously over the back of the piece of paper, and stuck it with force to the door on my way out.

Still fuming, I drove back as fast as I could in my little Fiat to the maternity ward that was at the far end of the vast hospital grounds. The facility had been built by the Italians when my husband, Mohamed Egal, was Prime Minister. I'd attended its grand opening and visited as First Lady. There were still photos of me hanging on the walls. Since 1972, I'd been a mere employee – the head of the maternity department until today, when I looked set to quit for the sake of a premature baby.

I didn't much care about the consequences at that point. I was far too weary to worry. I'd empty my desk and walk away. After all, what more could the regime do to me? They'd already taken my home and my belongings; they'd broken up my marriage;

they'd imprisoned, harassed and interrogated both my husband and me. They'd even shot my beloved cheetah. My only concern was for the three-day-old girl fighting for her life in an incubator.

I hurried to the ward where the baby's mother was waiting anxiously for news. Her hands in supplication, she asked, 'Will they send more oxygen?'

I shrugged. 'I don't honestly know, but let's prepare to take your baby to the Martini Hospital just in case. The doctors there won't let your daughter die.'

Before we could unplug the machine and wrap the baby in a blanket with a portable oxygen mask, a breathless soldier appeared carrying the cylinder I'd requested. 'The director sent me,' he said, wiping the sweat from his brow as he put down the heavy canister.

'About time,' I said, pointing to where I needed it to be rolled so that I could connect it to the machine. 'You can tell him from me that he must never, ever refuse me anything like this again. This oxygen isn't for me, it is for a sick little baby and I never want to fight about this again.'

The soldier agreed to carry my message but then stood around sheepishly.

'Yes?'

'The director says to tell you one last thing,' he added, looking ready to make a run for it. 'He asks that next time you promise not to use Superglue.'

Turning away to hide my smile, I nodded and waved him away.

Erigavo, British Somaliland, 1950

It was twenty-five years earlier, in the Year of Red Dust, known as *Siigacaase*, that my journey to nursing really began. The April rains in our part of Africa had failed again and the desert winds had dried the land to a powdered rust that choked and stifled. We were well accustomed to the dry season or *jiilal* from December to March each year; it was a time of thirst and suffering. In this our worst drought in years, though, more than seventy per cent of the livestock had perished and our nomadic people were penniless and starving.

I would turn thirteen that autumn, but even at such a tender age I saw for myself what famine and malnutrition did to the human body. As the eldest daughter of Adan Ismail – the most senior Somali medical professional in the country and its so-called 'Father of Healthcare' – I accompanied him every day of that long, hot summer to the forty-bed hospital where he worked tirelessly to treat people and try to save lives. Hour after hour I'd follow him on his rounds, taking instructions to feed a weak child or making sure that an elderly patient had their saline drip renewed. I cut up old sheets for bandages, washed syringes, and sterilized instruments long blunted. Although the city of Erigavo was the capital of the Sanaag region and part of the British Somaliland Protectorate, it was – as Dad said – 'too far from the cooking pot' – which translated to limited supplies and little support from the authorities based in Hargeisa.

As the man in charge of health services for the entire region, my father often had to leave town and drive long distances alone in his ex-British Army Bedford ambulance to tend to destitute families in the outlying refugee camps. In his absence he had no choice but to entrust the running of his hospital to the largely illiterate auxiliaries, only a few of whom were qualified. Fearing for his patients, he'd ask me to oversee them until his return. I was still only a child but his hospitals had always been my playground and I knew my way around. Whenever he was away, he'd leave me little notes telling me what to do so that I wouldn't forget. 'Make sure they remove the catheter from that patient tomorrow, Shukri,' he'd say using the name only he called me. Or he'd remind me, 'That mother's sutures need to come out on Monday... and don't forget to change the dressings on the child with burns in Ward 3.'

Known to all as 'Adan Dhakhtar', my father had been trained as a medical assistant by the British in the Crown Colony of Aden before the Second World War, and then later in England. He'd hoped to become a doctor, but a medical degree was never open to someone like him because it would have taken too long and cost the British taxpayer too much money. Instead, he was sent back to his country to take on the full responsibilities of a doctor (on a fraction of the salary), in a series of postings around the country that generally only lasted two years before he was moved on to a new home and a new hospital and new patients to treat. In each new city he was expected to do all this seven days a week and run an entire hospital compound in a role designated as a Compounder.

Far more revered than any British doctor and a versatile all-rounder, Dad treated every patient he encountered– no matter how poor, dirty, smelly or sick – with the utmost dignity and respect. I remember being enlisted by him once to hold a bowl under the face of a hawk-faced old man with an infected abscess in his jaw. The patient was elderly and unclean and my disgust at the pus my father lanced must have shown in my expression because once the old man had been cleaned up and left the room, Dad closed the door and turned on me.

'Don't you ever show such an ugly face to any of my patients again!' he said, his eyes flashing. 'If you cannot show respect, then stay away from this hospital.' His reprimand marked me for life and was my first important lesson in nursing care. It was then that I fell in love with medicine. The dirty old nomad was more precious to Adan Doctor than me, his first-born. To this day, if I see something smelly or disgusting or oozing I make a point of diving right in with both hands. It's my way of training my students that a nurse has to do whatever it takes and treat everyone with the same respect and care.

My father worked seven days a week, 365 days a year, and he loved every minute. Adan Ismail was my hero. He still is. I will never be as compassionate as he was. I will never be as kind and generous as he was with his time, his emotions, and his affection. My father was a very good man. Every day he was hindered by a chronic lack of funds and supplies, many of which he ended up paying for himself. And yet every day he still put on his uniform and went to work with a smile on his face. My mother used to call him 'the man with holes in the palms of his hands' because money slipped through them, usually spent on his hospital or his patients. Every day he'd say, 'If only I had more medicines', or 'I wish I had a better sterilizer.' He'd have happily bought these things himself but they weren't easily available in our forgotten part of Africa, so he was forever asking me to wash a pair of scissors or some other instrument because he didn't have enough or the quality was too poor. 'Not those ones,' he'd say, gently. 'They don't cut well. Bring me the others.' I wished I could have bought him a whole tray of sharp scissors, a box of gleaming new scalpels, or a pair of forceps that actually worked.

Watching him deal with these challenges every day planted a fertile seed inside my head: a quite fantastical thought for any little girl, but especially one growing up in a developing country. I can't recall the exact moment when I decided that I would one day build him a hospital, but I do know I had a very clear idea of how it would be run. My only image of the outside was that it was large and white, but I never sketched out any drawings or plans. My dream had much more to do with it being the right kind of place – a perfect new medical centre that would do my father proud. In my head it had all the equipment, instruments and trained staff that he'd need. It was a place where he would be delighted to work. And where I would happily work alongside him.

Back in 1950, my fantasy was little more than a child's wish to please her beloved father. It was far from realistic in a Muslim country that didn't even allow schooling for girls. Education for girls was unavailable in case we dared form any opinions or – worse – voice them. Anyway, there was little point when every Somali woman was expected to be a dutiful wife and mother, bound by archaic social traditions as well as often harmful traditional practices. Dad never saw me that way. I was his adored Shukri, his first child and one of three to survive out of five. He called me the 'apple of his eye' and encouraged me to read English from an early age. It was he who arranged for me to go to school in French Somaliland, determined that I should have the kind of opportunities he'd been given as a child. Like me, he dreamed that I would one day train as a nurse and help him offer the kind of healthcare he longed to provide for the people he loved. My father wanted me to be the best I could possibly be.

If I were to fulfil that wish then what better gift could I give him than his own hospital? How I would achieve it, I didn't know. What money I'd use to make it happen, I had no idea. Neither of us knew that political turmoil and civil war would soon devastate our country. We could never have foreseen the suffering. At twelve years old, I only knew that one day my father's name would be placed for all to see on a large white hospital built in his honour. I didn't even tell him of my secret plan. Yet the idea sprang into my young head so clear and bright and certain. It lodged in my subconscious like tumbleweed caught on a thorn, and that's where it remained for more than fifty years until I finally had the time and resources to do something about it. This is the story of how I made that happen, against insurmountable odds.

CHAPTER ONE

Hargeisa, British Somaliland Protectorate, 1937

Seven days after I was born at 9 p.m. on 8 September 1937 following a long and difficult delivery, my father gave me the name 'Shukri', which means thanks. This was because I was considered something of a miracle after two years of my mother's infertility.

The only reason I know the date of my birth is because I was born in a hospital in Hargeisa, unlike the majority of Somalilanders. We didn't mark birthdays in the same way as people in the West because we didn't then have a written language, very few people could read, and no one knew what a calendar was. Many my age don't know when they were born and say simply 'the time of bad floods', or 'the month before the long drought'. Age was counted by the rainy seasons, of which there are two, so a child who has seen two rains would be described as two years old when they were really only one.

I was a big, healthy baby although I carry two scars on my head from the forceps used by the English obstetrician who delivered me. Perhaps the miracle of my survival in a country where infant mortality is still the fourth highest in the world is the reason I became such a headstrong child and a stubborn adult – to which many will attest. With ninety-four in every 1,000 babies dying at birth in Somaliland (compared with four or five in the UK and the US), it is customary for newborns never to be named until they are a week old for fear their parents become too emotionally attached.

At my naming ceremony on 15 September, my mother Marian, a Somali who'd been raised a Catholic, called me Edna in honour of a Greek girlfriend who insisted that if I was a girl then I should take her name. It was a moniker Dad never once used. My arrival ended what my mother feared was a curse against her ever since she'd married my father two years earlier. Many of those who liked my father disapproved of his marriage and believed that he should have chosen a Muslim wife. This view only gained currency when Mum hadn't yet borne him a child, as, in our culture, it is normal for a wife to conceive straight away. If she doesn't it is usually blamed on 'the evil eye' or some other bad spirit and Allah is prayed to, so when Mum finally became pregnant with me the evil eye was considered to have blinked.

My father was over six feet tall, charismatic, generous, fluent in several languages and the best doctor and communicator I've ever met. To him, teaching people about healthcare was not only a duty but also a pleasure, and he threw his heart and soul into educating anyone he came across. One of his favourite expressions was, 'If you cannot do it with your heart then your hands will never learn to do it.'

His own father, Ismail Guleed, was something of a legend in Somaliland. A successful, silver-haired merchant from the noble Arap Isaaq clan of nomadic warriors and camel herders, he was known as Ismail *Gaado Cadde,* which means White Chest. This referred to the white hair on his chest that spilled over his tunic.

Wealth in my country is measured in camels – a female and her calf can cost £1,000 in today's terms – and my grandfather exported large herds of them. Independently wealthy, he hired traditional *dhow* boats to carry goods destined for Ethiopia and service his lucrative contract to supply livestock, firewood and ghee to the British garrison in the Aden Colony, sixty kilometres across the Gulf of Aden – the gateway to the Red Sea.

Grandfather Ismail naturally expected that his two sons – my uncle Mohamed and my father Adan, born in 1906 – would help run his business. He and his wife Baada had moved to Aden once their sons were of school age specifically so that they could be educated at St Joseph's, a Roman Catholic Mission School, the only place in the region where they could learn to read and write in English. Little did he know that my uncle Mohamed would jump on a ship bound for the Indian Ocean aged sixteen to become a merchant seaman for the rest of his life, while my father would choose medicine. Sadly, Grandfather died in his early sixties, so I never knew him. After his death my father tried to keep the family business going but it became too difficult to manage on top of his medical duties.

I sorely wished I'd asked Dad what made him decide to study medicine because it was truly a vocation for him and something he dedicated his whole life to. Perhaps there was an incident that inspired him. As far as I'm aware, he was never ill, but he did have multiple scars on his legs from playing football and hockey so perhaps that was how he encountered the miracle of medicine.

★★★

My earliest childhood memories are of my grandmothers' faces, fleeting images of their beaming smiles. These women were perhaps the most influential in my immediate family, although the men in our vast extended clan traditionally exerted the most control. As another Somali girl child my infancy was rather uneventful, apart from the day I disappeared as a baby. Mum left me sleeping on her bed with cushions stacked all around me to prevent me from falling off, then went to the outdoor kitchen at the back of our house to prepare lunch – probably *sabaya* flatbreads with some curry or beans and rice. Our single-storey detached house had two bedrooms as well as a living/dining room. There was no flushing toilet, just a shaded pit latrine in the yard, and my mother, the cook and a maid heated water over firewood laid on stones and cooked meat over a charcoal burner made from oil drums.

When my mother came to check on me a little while later, she found me missing and the pillows undisturbed. Perplexed, she thought my father must have come home from the hospital in his break and carried me outside. When she couldn't find us in the yard, she believed he'd taken me back to his hospital without telling her. In a country with regular epidemics of smallpox and other diseases she, like most Somali women of her generation, had a terrible fear of taking a healthy child to a place full of sick people so – furious – she hurried to the hospital only to find Dad alone. He was just as surprised to see her because she never visited unless for a medical emergency. Mum immediately started wailing that I had been stolen. They hurried back home and they, the servants, our neighbours, and eventually the police looked frantically for me and traces of my 'kidnapper'. Amidst the hubbub, no one thought to look under our dining room table to which I had crawled beneath the tablecloth to resume my nap. Once I was discovered my mother never lived down the embarrassment and Dad would often tell me how lucky I was that I wasn't chained to the bed after that.

I was only two when the Italians declared war on the Allies in June 1940 and in August invaded British Somaliland and Ethiopia.

I have no recollection of the events of the Second World War or the impact upon our family. Nor do I recall the events just before that when my mother's next child, my unnamed infant sister, died a few minutes after birth following another harrowing forceps delivery. Mum was frail and still recovering when the British declared that all the wives and children of civil servants should evacuate to a small fishing village on the Gulf of Aden. From there we'd board a British naval destroyer for Aden.

My grandmother Clara, my mother's mother, supervised everything. As they were only allowed to take minimal luggage she wrapped cash, jewellery and the family's most precious things in a bag she tied around her waist. In the fishing village we were placed in different huts to await the signal that the warship had arrived in the dead of night. My mother, grandmother and I were shivering together in one such hut with several others when a band of thieves burst in brandishing knives and demanding valuables. Clara quickly blew out the kerosene lamp, which plunged the hut into darkness. The women started screaming, which alerted the local villagers who arrived just as the robbers fled. Many claimed afterwards that if it wasn't for my grandmother they'd have lost everything they possessed.

Once in Aden, Clara once again took charge, selling possessions to rent us a comfortable property. She and my mother had no idea what had happened to my father and grandfather, who'd remained behind to serve the Allies. It was months before we learned that they'd been captured and imprisoned by the Italians and packed into cells in a makeshift prisoner-of-war camp in Hargeisa. Dad spoke of his experiences later and told me that they were treated badly, with little food or water and no toilet facilities. Their cell was hot and crowded with nowhere to sit. 'If you ever have to go to prison be sure to take a hat with you, Shukri,' he advised.

'To urinate we'd stand on each other's backs and pee out of the window, but the only receptacle we had for bigger business was a fellow prisoner's hat!'

Hargeisa had fallen to the Italians on 5 August 1940, despite repeated RAF sorties that dropped more than sixty tons of bombs on Somaliland. The rest of the country fell two weeks later with the loss of thirty-eight Allied soldiers and more than two hundred wounded. It was another few months before the operation to recapture it began in early 1941. Hargeisa was liberated – along with my father and grandfather – and the famous Somaliland Camel Corps (a British Army unit based in Somaliland) resumed its military operations. The Italians were pushed out and we were free to go home.

Once back home, my parents discovered that although our government-owned house was still standing, it had been ransacked and the looters had done more damage than the shelling. Hargeisa Hospital, which was erected by the British military during the Second World War and initially comprised mostly tents, had been partly damaged too, so Dad lived in quarters until my mother could get things straight at home. Many friends and relatives had been killed or injured and the only event that brightened our lives was the birth of my brother in late 1941. Farah was born prematurely and was more than four years my junior, but he became my joy as well as the pride of our family.

★★★

Having survived the Italians my first proper memories are of Berbera, a major coastal town we lived in until I was six years old and where the smell of the ocean pervaded everything. A key character in those recollections was a man known as 'Mohammed

Hindi' or Mohammed the Indian who ran a *dukaan* or general store on a corner not far from where we lived. In it, he sold every kind of foodstuff.

As Somali women didn't often leave their homes, Dad did most of the shopping and would often take me with him as a treat. Mohammed would see me and, with a huge grin, cry, 'Ah! A biscuit for the doctor's daughter!' before handing me a custard cream from a counter cluttered with sweets. Nothing has ever tasted as nice before or since even though I have had them in every country I have visited; I am still looking for the divine taste of *those* old-fashioned British custard creams. My second big treat in that corner shop was to be allowed to stir the ice cream while Dad shopped for the weekly provisions of sugar, rice, flour, corned beef, tins of beans, butter and jam. Mohammed made the ice cream in a huge bowl packed in blocks of ice, adding eggs, milk, sugar and cardamom that had to be churned the old-fashioned way. If I was lucky, he'd also let me lick the bowl.

I remember that wooden shack of a store so clearly with its high tin roof and dry goods piled to the rafters. It was in the area of town where the Europeans lived, so the shopkeeper cleverly catered to their needs with foreign goods. To me, it seemed as if he sold every item in the world stacked haphazardly, and yet he knew exactly where everything was. I loved that kind, smiling Indian and I loved being spoiled, much to the consternation of my mother Marian. She was, I think, disappointed in me her whole life. From the day I crawled under the dining room table to my later more controversial years I was trouble in her eyes. From the outset I was a rebellious child, devoted to my father, and favoured by both grandmothers. My *hooyo* (mother), expected me to stay inside and do household chores such as peel potatoes, prepare onions or help wash the sheets. I hated such tasks and would much rather play barefoot outside with my pets, seek out wild animals, climb a tree, or wrestle with the neighbourhood boys. The only job I did enjoy was to accompany the house help down to the well by the river to refill the empty water barrels, something he did at least twice a day. Whenever he had to stop and rest in the heat as he rolled the filled barrel back up the hill to replenish our tank, I had to wedge a large stone under it to stop it rolling away. This felt to me like important, valuable work.

I once found a snake in our household water tank and spent ages trying to get it out with a stick, but was roundly scolded by my mother who was terrified I'd be bitten. Mum kept insisting that I needed to be trained as to how a Somali girl should be correctly brought up. She bought me pretty dresses that were quickly ruined and did her best to tame my Afro hair, tugging at it with a wide-toothed comb until I screamed, or trying to twist it into plaits which quickly came undone. Whenever I was made to stay inside with her, I showed such little aptitude for cooking or sewing that she'd soon release me from my chore. Sulking I'd sit on the verandah peering out and measuring the time of day by the *eedhaan*, the traditional call to prayer at dawn, midday, mid-afternoon, dusk and at night. If I was really bored I'd flick through my parents' precious English books wondering what the strange symbols meant, only to be accused of ruining them with dirty fingers when I had no business looking at them, being an 'illiterate girl'.

I loved it best when Dad came home from work at the end of the day and sat to eat with us by the light of a kerosene lamp as giant moths flapped noisily at the mosquito screens. He'd instruct that the fire be lit on cold nights and burned frankincense to fill the house with the heavenly scent that is thought to be spiritually healing and chase away evil spirits. Sadly, Dad worked so hard that he never seemed to have time to linger, running back to the hospital at the slightest emergency after a hug and a kiss. He was an unusually affectionate man in a society where men are not supposed to show affection in case it's seen as a sign of weakness. My father loved my mother very much and put up with a lot from her. The youngest and most spoilt of two daughters raised in Aden by Somali parents who were from a small community of Catholics, she was more English than the Queen in many ways and always envisaged a better life. Her sister Cecilia had married a successful businessman from French Somaliland and the couple had moved there to raise a family. By marrying a Muslim and remaining in Somaliland, my mother had tied herself to a life that dictated she should have little of any importance to occupy her days. I know she loved my father very much and it can't have been easy married to a workaholic who was moved from town to town every two years, but she was often depressed and never stopped complaining.

From an early age I began to appreciate that boys and girls were different, and by that I mean that girls only ever played in small groups in their own homes or back yards up until the age of about eight and the older ones were rarely spotted outside. Instead they were expected to remain inside learning how to be a good wife. That wasn't for me, so I had no choice but to play on my own until my father erected a long rope swing in our yard, the only one in the neighbourhood, to which local boys would flock. I loved running around with these fellow children of government officials. One of these was Hassan Abdillahi Walanwal Kayd, who was two or three years older than me, taller and more handsome than the others, and one of those I was determined to keep up with. Little did I know then how our paths would collide for much of my life.

Unfortunately, most of them were embarrassed to be seen play-ing with a girl and chased me away whenever I tried to join in. The only exception was when it came to foraging. Near our house was a little garden that surrounded the grave of some prominent person, and it had a mighty gob tree. *Gob* means noble and these noble trees not only look majestic but give us shade, food, shelter and wood. The yellow berries are like sweet little cherries so the boys and I would clamber over the wall and throw stones to bring down those delicious fruits.

Neighbours and relatives would often complain to my mother that they had seen me running barefoot in the sandy streets again. 'How can you allow that, Marian?' they'd berate. 'It's not proper. A girl isn't brought up to run wild outside and play with boys.' But my mother couldn't control me and my father didn't intend to. Mum would simply chastise me constantly with, 'Where have you been, Edna?' Or, 'Where are you going now? Playing with the boys again, I suppose? Ugh. Well, at least put on some shoes!' I hated wearing shoes and one of my arguments against them was that spiders and scorpions frequently crawled inside so I was safer without. This meant that my feet were permanently dirty and grazed (along with my knees) and a daily pastime was asking my mother or a servant to pull acacia thorns from my soles.

The neighbourhood girls who'd heard their mothers complain about my inappropriate behaviour soon followed suit, insultingly calling me a '*wiilo*', which means tomboy. My response was to fight them, which only got me into more trouble. If I couldn't play with the boys I'd go off exploring and looking for animals in the thorn bushes, only returning to the house to eat some papaya, help myself to some *tiin* or prickly pear from the yard, or to water from the tank. Nature had always fascinated me and I knew every little lizard, squirrel, frog, rabbit or beetle that lived around our property. On hot languid days in the dry season I liked to sit in the shade of a tree, inhaling the scent of jasmine and listening to the chatter of the yaryaro birds. When it was cooler I'd chase the mini tornados known as sand devils that danced down our street. I was repeatedly warned against the hyenas that came at night looking for food, and wasn't supposed to stray too far.

My parents never once gave me any pocket money to spend but they did buy me toys, usually blonde blue-eyed dolls, which were fun for a short while. I also had a wooden camel on wheels made by a kind British carpenter. I soon grew tired of these playthings, though, because they didn't move or interact like my cat or my pet goat Orggi or the wild creatures out in the yard. Something that amused me for hours was making drinking glasses from empty bottles, and little lanterns out of old Player's cigarettes tins, with a kerosene-soaked wick stuffed inside and a hole in the lid for it to poke through. There were severe shortages after the war and many household items were no longer available in the market, so we learned to improvise. The lanterns were easy to make but their wicks smelled even more noxious than the usual paraffin lamps and were a fire hazard, plus they stained Mum's white walls with black smoke. I much preferred these kinds of activities to peeling onions or potatoes or beating the dust from the rugs.

From the earliest age I longed for a sibling and, although I was thrilled when my brother Farah arrived, I was crushed when I realized that he was too little to play with. Then my mother fell pregnant again. It is only with the wisdom of hindsight that I have come to understand why she chose to have this child at home with a traditional 'midwife' rather than in the safety of a hospital run by her husband. In spite of her cosmopolitan upbringing, in the nine years since her marriage to my father she'd remodelled herself into the archetypal Somali housewife who kept close counsel with her female friends and took too great a heed of their scaremongering. 'Don't tell your husband when you go into labour,' they warned her. 'He will only take you to hospital and put things inside you. The British doctors already killed one daughter and put a scar on Edna's face. Call us instead. We'll bring the midwife and she'll help you deliver naturally at home.'

The morning that Mum's waters broke she didn't say a word to Dad as he completed his customary 6 a.m. ablutions, shaved, and slicked back his hair. As the head of the household, he always had priority in the bathroom. While experiencing labour pains, she cooked his *laxoox* pancakes made from sorghum flour for breakfast, which we smothered in ghee, honey or jam. She waited for him to dress in his regulation white shorts, white shirt, white socks and polished shoes, knowing that he would then walk to work to arrive punctually at 7 a.m. His hospital was really only a series of Army tents around two brick buildings, one of which was the operating theatre, but whenever I could, I'd walk with Dad all the way down the sandy street to the hospital gate, immensely proud of the meticulously dressed man holding my hand who commanded so much respect in our community. The only thing that would tempt me to break from his side was if I saw the local boys running somewhere, then I'd kiss him goodbye and hurtle off in their direction while he laughed.

Back at home that morning, my mother's labour pains intensified so she summoned her girlfriends as instructed and they called an *umulisso*, an elderly woman known as a 'traditional midwife' who had no nursing training or qualifications. The servants kept me out of the way as I listened in horror to my mother wailing and grunting for hours, wondering what on earth they were doing to her. The 'midwife' finally delivered Mum of a healthy baby boy, but then accidentally dropped the slippery baby, killing him instantly when he landed on his head. I was six years old and will never forget my mother's screams. The women tried to calm her as the midwife wrapped her otherwise perfect baby boy in the tiny blanket that would become his shroud.

'He's so beautiful!' I declared, when I crept into the room and stood over the tiny body in the crib, not much bigger than my doll. 'Can I keep him?' Someone pushed me out of the room and told a servant to run to the hospital and tell my father the news. The message Dad received was, 'Come home and bury your son.' In the Muslim faith, a body is buried within twenty-four hours of death. As my father knew nothing of the birth he immediately assumed that Farah had been killed in an accident and half-expected to find his mangled body. Running home, a thousand possibilities raced through his mind, he was overwhelmed with relief when – in a house of weeping women – he discovered Farah alive and well, but then shattered to learn that the infant son he didn't know he had was dead because of the carelessness of an untrained woman.

At such a tender age, I was appalled at the idea of my baby brother being taken away to be buried in the ground, and created quite a scene at the house. 'Why do you have to take him? Don't take him away! I want to keep him!' I cried, until my grandmother Baada pulled me away and the burial proceeded as planned.

My paternal grandmother Baada was kindness itself and I learned so much from her. She was an eloquent woman who taught me my first words and the names of plants, as well as songs, rhymes and stories. She lived close by all her life and would come to our house every morning, bringing me treats she hid from my mother. One look at her face and I'd know she was carrying something – most likely sweets made out of caramel with lumps of sugar and nuts. She also taught me how to be curious, offering me a choice between something I knew or something I didn't. I'd almost always opt for the thing I didn't know. I still do.

My disapproving mother frequently guessed that she had given me something and would protest, but I didn't care. I loved my grandmother. We had a conspiracy together behind my mother's back. It was our little secret. What I didn't yet know was how many other secrets there were in female Somali society, the darkest of which was being kept from me.

CHAPTER TWO

Borama, British Somaliland, 1945

Some of my happiest childhood memories are of drinking fresh cow's milk during our long summer holidays in Borama, near the border with Ethiopia, where my grandmother Clara and grandfather Yusuf lived. I remember going with the maid to collect the frothy warm nectar from Granddad's cows and helping myself to as much as I liked. I'm sure my father would have disapproved. He always insisted – as I do now – that any milk intended for his children had to be boiled first to avoid contamination. To this day, though, and even after all my years of training as a nurse and public health practitioner, I occasionally sneak a drink of fresh, unboiled camel milk.

The reason we spent so much time in Borama in the north-western Awdal province was because the British had posted my grandfather there after the Italians left Somaliland. Having trained as a signalman and radio operator Yusuf had served the British in both wars and was awarded a military medal for 'meritorious service to the Crown'. Then he became Somaliland's Postmaster-General. Although our country was liberated, the war was still raging elsewhere and his expertise in logistics was needed to facilitate the East Africa Campaign. He soon fell in love with the lush green meadows of Borama fringed by purple mountains and decided to buy a farm and some milking cows, summoning Clara to join him.

My mother would leave us with our grandparents for two months each summer so that she could visit friends in Aden, or her sister Cecilia in Djibouti City in French Somaliland. She may have become a good Muslim and embraced all the traditions and rituals, but she sorely missed the country and lifestyle of her childhood in Aden. Sending us away each year must have been a welcome respite from the nuisance I'd become. Not that I was any less of a problem for my grandparents. Borama was a holiday town and kids from all over Somaliland and from Djibouti City descended for the summer months. I sometimes hung out with girls, but it was still the company of boys that I liked the best. When one time the local gang wouldn't let me play football with them I retaliated by snatching their ball made of bound rags and ran home with it. I locked myself in the toilet and threatened to throw their ball into the pit unless they agreed to let me join in. My mother was still there then and she had to intervene. After much pleading, she got me to open the door and give back the ball. From then on, one of the boys would grab it whenever I approached their game, afraid that I'd snatch it once more.

One day these boys came to me with an unusual gesture of friendship and asked if I wanted to join them. This was too good to be true and I jumped at the chance. A few minutes after our game of football started on a patch of waste ground, they told me they were going to pick some watermelons from a nearby field and that if I helped carry some home, we'd return to our game sooner. Naturally I agreed, hoping that I'd finally been accepted. I innocently followed them through a gap in a fence and offered to carry the largest of the watermelons in my upturned skirt, as it was too heavy to carry in my arms. As I was tottering back with a fruit that weighed almost as much as I did, the farmer suddenly grabbed me by the scruff of my dress.

The boys melted away, leaving me to face the irate landowner who marched me back to my grandparents' house carrying the melon as proof of my guilt. I tried to explain and swore that I'd never stolen anything, but my grandparents almost died of shame. When he complained that kids trespassed almost daily to help themselves to his crop, they had no option but to compensate him for the loss of God knows how many melons he claimed I'd taken. The disappointment on my grandparents' faces was worse than any punishment they could have meted out. I had to listen to them telling me over and over that they couldn't understand why I'd steal when everything I could want to eat was available on our own table.

In spite of this salutary lesson, as the oldest in our group of neighbourhood friends and the big sister to Farah, I was the Pied Piper for all our adventures. These included the time a group of us unknowingly picked poisonous berries and all returned home with swollen lips. I took the blame for not supervising the others carefully enough, and from then on we weren't allowed to eat anything we picked until we'd brought it home for adults to inspect and either confirm or confiscate.

Then there was the day that nine of us wandered into the bush and completely lost our way. Boy, I never lived that one down. Even though we'd eaten a full breakfast, we always had room for delicious wild berries. As we picked more and more, we wandered near the path of the donkey caravans on their way to collect water at the wells on the outskirts of town. The herders instantly identified us as town kids because of the way we dressed, and were surprised to find us still in the forest several hours later when they returned.

Seeing that some of the younger ones were crying, and others had slumped down through exhaustion and thirst, they stopped to ask what we were doing there so late in the afternoon. 'Who brought you here? Why aren't you at home?' they asked, clearly concerned. I told them that although I knew where the sun rose and set, I couldn't tell in the woods and none of us had a clue how to get back to town. With night falling and knowing that hyenas or lions could start to pick us off, the donkey herders scooped up the youngest children and sat them on their beasts while telling we older ones to walk fast, stick together, and follow their caravan. We trudged along the dusty track used by generations of nomads, past colonies of noisy baboons, and finally reached town just before sunset. We found the whole district in a state of panic, and distressed parents who'd been searching everywhere for us berated me. 'How could you be so stupid to stray so far?' As the eldest child, I was given the harshest scolding but the worst punishment was that our neighbours warned their kids never to follow 'crazy Edna' again if I ever tried to lead them beyond the trees they then set as landmarks at the edge of the forest.

Despite these occasional mishaps, Farah and I loved it in Borama far from the heat of a city, especially when we were able to have as much fresh milk as we liked. My grandmother made the most delicious butter, boiling the milk then skimming off the cream and churning it just like Mohammed the Indian had done with ice cream. When she wasn't cooking or caring for us, Clara worked in the local hospital, interpreting for the English-speaking medical staff, so I would happily tag along with her in her long Somali dress, eager to hear their cries when we approached of 'Ayeeyo timid!' (Grandma is here!). I watched as she'd sit with the patients before translating for the staff. It was painstaking work but she was caring, kind and gentle. How could I not go into medicine with such remarkable role models?

Her only sadness, I think, was the way my grandfather treated her. She was unusually meek in his presence and still he picked on her. He'd complain, 'Why is lunch cold?' or 'Where's my coat, woman?' My mother took after him far more than she did Clara. If ever I had a problem, I'd go to my grandmother, who was my ally and my friend.

★★★

Coming from a household of two different religions was an interesting experience for a child. My father was very religious and at every call to prayer he would stop what he was doing to kneel on his mat. He also attended the mosque every Friday and, as a family, we marked Ramadan and Eid.

My grandparents – and occasionally my mother – would go to mass, sing hymns and receive a blessing from the priest, and we also celebrated Christmas and Easter, showing respect for all. Then for the Islamic feasts the cook Ali would slaughter a sheep and people would come to our house to help break the fast. My father was always extremely generous to those who had less than us and usually invited six or seven poor families to take away packages of meat, dates and bread – food many of them came to rely on.

One day when we were expecting guests for lunch, I came upon Ali about to carve up my pet goat Orggi, which he'd already caught and slaughtered. When I became hysterical and tried to stop him, he told me that my kid was to be cooked for the feast. I was eventually pulled away from the scene kicking and screaming, but continued to howl until Dad came home. 'They killed my friend and are going to feed him to the guests!' I wailed. Goodness alone knows what he thought. In spite of his attempts to comfort me, I couldn't understand how Dad could allow them do such a thing to my playmate. I never got over it.

Even though my father worked every day and stayed late, people who needed him out of hours would still seek him out, so there was often someone knocking at the door with a problem. No matter if he was hungry and about to put a spoon to his mouth, if someone called he'd put it down, rise from his chair and tend to their needs. My mother hated that. She often claimed that the hospital was his first wife and that he spent more time there than with us. 'Where are you running off to again? Why even bother to come home?' she'd say, or ask, 'Why do you have to do this? Why can't someone else do it?' She considered the patients who called at our house trespassers on our privacy and complained bitterly that this was our home, not a hospital. 'Besides, what if one of them brings disease into our house?' she'd cry, exasperated.

Dad never argued with her and tried to explain that people couldn't help it if they got sick at all times of the day and night. He was passionate about his work and he loved to be needed. With an open face and an open heart, smiling and happy, he'd never turn someone away or tell them, 'I'm too busy, come and see me tomorrow.' Instead, he'd sit and listen to their problems. My father was just as generous with his money. There were so many people on his list of charitable donations each month that he must surely have lost count. People I thought were relatives often turned out to be the orphans of a school friend or the wife of a football teammate who was on hard times whose bills were being paid for by Dad.

Everyone assumed he was extremely wealthy, which only led to more name calling by some of the kids in my neighbour-hood, who'd say, 'Why do you want to play with us, rich girl?' I remember running home to ask my mother what their insult meant. She explained that we weren't as poor as many others, adding somewhat bitterly that we'd be even richer if my father wasn't quite so generous with our money.

In the same magnanimous way, Dad decided to help improve the education of some local boys and our younger male cousins by hiring a teacher to come to our house every afternoon, except Friday. These boys already attended the local school – forbidden for girls – but the teaching there was limited and Dad hoped to expand their horizons. He paid for a blackboard, chalk and textbooks, and set everything up on our verandah where the pupils squatted on the cement floor with their books on their knees. Many of them were the boys I tagged along with, including Hassan Kayd, so whenever they stopped kicking an old tennis ball around in the dust to hurry to lessons at my house, I would follow. I think now that this was my father's intention all along.

It was for me to choose whether to carry on playing outside or be curious enough to see what the boys were doing. He knew I had an enquiring mind and hoped that this would pull me in the right direction. So, from the age of six or seven I'd sit on the edge of the verandah listening in or writing out my alphabet as I learned English, how to do calculations, and discovered a bit more about the world. The teacher never told me that I couldn't be there, but if I ever tried to answer a question he'd shush me and tell me not to interfere. I knew my place; I was allowed to stay because it was my father's house but I couldn't take part – even if I knew more of the answers than the rest. My mother didn't mind me joining in either because it meant a couple of hours' peace, and stopped me from running wild in the streets.

Those lessons were such a revelation to me. In a colonial region where people spoke and wrote in either Arabic, English, Italian or French, we Somalis didn't yet have a written language of our own, just an oral one. It seemed like magic then that I could put letters from the English alphabet together to make a word, and then words together to make a sentence. Newly inspired, I'd pick up a book from my father's bookcase and flick through the pages looking for a 'T' or an 'S' and then – oh my gosh – there they were! Every day brought a new discovery and I remember the moment I spelled out the word for cat, and was so excited because I had one of those. Reading opened up the miracle of forming something meaningful in my head. I'd always spoken a little English, but now I was able to decipher the mysteries of the alphabet and the secret language between my parents.

'Could you leave me some M-O-N-E-Y before you go?' Mum would ask my dad, and I could finally understand what she was asking for. Enthused with my newfound knowledge, I began to read my mother's *Illustrated London News*, *Woman*, and *Woman's Own* magazines, which had to be read with the greatest care and passed on unspoiled to the next woman whose name was listed on the cover. I loved those 1940s magazines with their Western fashions, hats and colourful clothes. The lives they depicted seemed like a million miles away from my own in hot, dusty Somaliland.

I wanted to read everything I could after that. I still do. My brain was hungry for knowledge and information. I needed to feed that hunger and when my parents saw me staring intently at the pages of a book, they asked what I was doing. 'Reading, of course,' I replied.

'Let's see what you're reading,' my father said, thinking I was just pretending but, to his amazement, he found that I *was* reading and learning to pronounce new words. There then began an ongoing family discussion about what to do with a girl who was teaching herself to read in a country where there were no schools for girls. Both my parents had been educated and recognized my yearning. After much debate, they decided to send me to a mission school. I think my mother hoped that the discipline would be the making of me, while my father hoped it would open the door to higher education and eventually nursing. Little did he know.

★★★

Djibouti City was four hundred kilometres away from Hargeisa, but it was the natural choice for my schooling rather than Aden because I could lodge with my Aunt Cecilia. Her businessman husband had been killed several years earlier in a road accident while she was pregnant with her fourth child. When the shipment he was transporting to Ethiopia was looted after the accident, she lost the income from it too. Widowed and penniless, she never remarried and single-handedly raised all her children – Rita, Sonny, Tony and Madeleine who were older than me but familiar from family visits.

The first I knew that I was going to be educated was when my parents asked me if I'd like to go home with my cousins after their summer holiday that year. It must have been 1945, and although the war was still going on elsewhere, our corner of Africa was safe.

'Really?' I asked, astonished.

'Yes, really,' my father confirmed. 'Well, you want to go to school, don't you?'

This momentous event happened in my eighth year, which proved to be the most significant of my entire life. Going to a proper school for the first time felt like such a milestone. I had never been out of Somaliland, so from the moment I left my eyes were like saucers at the wonder of it all. To make ends meet, Aunt Cecilia worked as a dressmaker and a teacher in a domestic science school. For extra income, she took me in and, later, my brother Farah. She also homed my cousins Gracie and her brother Maurice – the motherless children of an uncle whose wife had died in childbirth – all of us sharing one large apartment that was permanently filled with music, chatter and noise. My aunt was a most resourceful woman and another powerful role model. She had the energy of twenty horses and her determination helped shape me.

Cecilia ran our lives like a military operation. Speaking only English and French so that I'd learn my two new languages quickly, she paired me up with the older kids to do chores such as polish our shoes and make our own beds. We sat at the big table in the living room to do our homework after school, and in the evenings we learned how to crochet or knit by the light of Tilley lamps. If we wanted her to make us something to wear then we had to hem it ourselves, sew the buttons on, and fold it neatly for her – or there would be no garment. My mother never taught me things like that, so I didn't take to everything at first but soon got the hang of it.

My first day at the École de la Nativité run by Franciscan nuns in white habits was overwhelming chiefly because it was full of white kids, and most of them boys. I had only ever seen one or two white people before – men who sometimes worked with Dad – but I don't think I'd ever seen white children. There must have been over a hundred pupils in the school – French, Somali, American, Italian, Greek, Jewish, Armenian, Ethiopian, and a few Arabs from Yemen. I was the only girl from Somaliland. Boys and girls sat together in the same class, a fact that further inflamed my relatives back in Somaliland who considered this lack of segregation scandalous. My mother Marian, already the target of their criticism, could only sigh and blame my father once more. How she must have longed for a 'normal' daughter who'd stay home, learn to cook, marry young and produce a healthy brood of grandchildren.

There was so much to take in at the École and my brain was like a sponge, soaking up everything. My cousin Madeleine, who was four years my senior (and my childhood heroine), attended the same school, so I didn't have to face it alone. The hardest thing to deal with was that overnight my world suddenly became French and I learned about Napoleon, Jeanne d'Arc, the three Louis' and Charlemagne in a language that was foreign to me. I studied the geography of France, recited the prayers of the French catechism and learned more about Islam. I was taught respect for all beings, all faiths. After a faltering start, I did well enough to jump up a year in my class and then again.

Life in Djibouti City opened up a whole new world to me. I couldn't wait to start my day and learn something new; I wanted to experience all that life had to offer. I was forever running around with loads of energy and few, if any, inhibitions. The nuns, each known as Sister (or in French *Soeur*) were all very different. I met one of them, Marie Thérèse who taught us maths and became Mother Superior, again in 1991 and asked if she remembered me. She grimaced, 'Of course, Edna – you were *toujours turbulente!*'

Little did she know just how turbulent I would become.

CHAPTER THREE

Hargeisa, British Somaliland, 1946

The summer of 1946 marked my first visit home after living in French Somaliland for one year. I was still only eight years old and little did I know that this would be the year that my life changed for ever. It felt good to be home as I had missed my grandmothers and my father especially. I couldn't wait to tell Dad my news and share all that I'd learned in school.

The strangest thing about being back was that I had a new perspective. My time in a French-run co-educational and largely secular environment had shown me that girls could participate in life as fully as boys, so to return to a place that put so many constraints on my gender felt all the more difficult to accept. None of the local girls I'd left behind were ever seen outside their homes and only the boys seemed to have any freedom – or fun. The camels had more freedom than we did.

When I was growing up I'd noticed something else unusual about the girls in our district. There was a mysterious event that made them disappear for a month or so and when they returned they were different – far more subdued and not participating as much as they'd done before. I thought that maybe they'd been ill and slow to recover, or that their mothers had warned them to behave in a more adult manner. Usually I was too busy playing with the boys to worry too much about why any one girl was acting strangely.

Circumcision for boys was an accepted part of our society, although I had little or no understanding of it. We'd often see the boys walk around gingerly afterwards in their *lunghis* or long overshirts, carefully holding the cloth away from their groins. As I had no knowledge of the human anatomy, periods or anything like that I didn't associate what had happened to them with their genitals. In any event, it was an unwritten rule in our society that we never discussed such matters. We girls were especially ignorant and blind so, despite being an inquisitive child, I knew nothing of the traditional rites and rituals because all that was one big secret.

One day that summer, I found myself alone in the house with my mother. My brother was in Borama visiting our grandparents and Dad was out of town visiting the nomads for a few days. These were people who'd often never seen a doctor in their lives and managed any health problems as best they could or with the ministrations of traditional herbalists, bone-setters and spiritual healers. The sick often fell prey to quack 'pharmacists' who sold them anything from pills to ward off the evil eye or an injection with something that could potentially be fatal. Whenever my father returned from these trips he'd be exhausted.

That particular morning after he'd left I awoke to find our house bustling with unusual commotion. For some reason, several women – cousins, neighbours, and relatives I called 'aunts' – had dropped in to talk with my mother and my Grandmother Baada. There was much hushed chatter and conversations clearly not meant for my ears. 'Why don't you go play outside?' Mum said when she caught me trying to listen in, and – although surprised – I was more than happy to oblige.

Early the following morning, one of my mother's friends turned up at the house with a strange old woman I'd never seen before, and a fattened sheep. These were only ever brought to the house for feast days and, as far as I knew, this wasn't one of them, so I was even more mystified. Odder still, Mum told me to take a shower, after which I assumed I'd be expected to put on my best clothes. 'No, no. Wear a clean nightdress,' she instructed. How peculiar, I thought. Equally strange, my bed was pushed into a corner of my bedroom and a mat laid on the floor. Someone placed a stool in the corridor and when I emerged from the shower room I found a group of women standing around it waiting for me. Smiling shyly at them, I wondered what was happening and then I realized with a pang of hunger that no one had prepared me any breakfast that morning.

No sooner had I sat down on the stool as instructed than mother's friends grabbed my arms while others yanked up my nightie, grabbed my legs and pulled them apart. One woman gripped my left leg and another my right, while a third held me in a stranglehold, pressing me down firmly by my shoulders. In a well-planned operation that relied on speed and surprise, I spotted a knife glinting in the morning light streaming through the window and screamed as the old woman squatted before me and started cutting between my legs.

I can still remember the pain more than seven decades later, and I live that moment over and over again each time I think about it. I could feel the knife slashing through the sensitive flesh of my private parts and the stickiness of my blood as I screamed and struggled. My mother and grandmother watched my ordeal but neither came to my rescue. They just stood there, ululating joyfully as they witnessed what we now call FGM, female genital mutilation – a barbaric, ritualistic circumcision far more common than vaccination in my country – designed to act as a human chastity belt until the night of my marriage.

I must have passed out because I can remember waking up physically and emotionally exhausted. I had no more fight left in me. There was a horrible wheezing sound coming from my throat. The next thing I knew, the old woman was stitching together my wound with acacia thorns, pulling them together with string like a shoelace. The pain was excruciating. In what felt like a living nightmare, my legs were then bound all the way up to the thighs and hips. The women then lifted me onto the disposable mat that would soak up my blood and had been laid on my bedroom floor for this purpose. It had been so carefully planned. The old woman sprinkled a mixture of herbs, sugar and a raw egg yolk onto my open wound to form some sort of crust.

'Egg will make you fertile,' she declared with a toothless smile. 'And sugar will make you sweet.' Now that I'm a nurse, I can't help but think that the mixture was a perfect medium to enable bacteria to grow, plastered onto an open wound by a woman with dirty hands, a dirty knife, using dirty rags. It was so gruesome at the time, and it is still gruesome to recall.

As I lay on the floor bleeding and sobbing in shock and pain, I was astonished that not one person showed me any sympathy at all. There was nobody to cry with or complain to, including my own flesh and blood. On the contrary, they were in a happy, festive mood. The sheep was slaughtered outside and a grand lunch prepared, with many of our neighbours summoned to share the special meal in my honour. The daughter of Adan Ismail had been 'cleansed' and all were invited to partake of the purification feast and celebrate the occasion. The women I loved the most in the world and who I'd always thought would protect me had deliberately selected the day for my *gudniin* or circumcision when they knew my father would be out of town. They then stood by while this horrific ritual was performed on me without any anaesthetic. They saw me kicking. They heard my screams. They paid for my butchery to be performed by someone who was neither medically qualified nor professionally trained.

They never warned me of what was about to happen in what I now understand to be a conspiracy of silence among Somali and other women dating back centuries. Far from being horrified at this brutal thing that had been done to me, they were happy and relieved about it.

As an eight-year old child, I could not comprehend it.

As a woman in her eighties, I still cannot accept it.

★★★

The next thing I really remember was hearing my father's voice. It must have been much later that night when he returned from the bush. Unable to move for the pain, I cried out to him. 'Daddy! My Daddy!' as he hurried in to see me.

Holding up a Tilley lamp, he took one look at me and fell to his knees, his prone figure casting a huge shadow on the wall. 'What have they done to you, Shukri? What have they done?'

My grandmother berated him from the doorway, telling him that it was nothing to do with him and that he shouldn't interfere. The women genuinely believed that if I were seen by a man then it could 'contaminate' my purification so that the wound wouldn't heal, the skin wouldn't fuse together, and the procedure might have to be done again. Ignoring his own mother, he slumped onto the mat and cradled me in his arms, allowing me to cry and cry until there were no more tears.

'Aabo wey i qasheen!' I wept. 'Father, they slaughtered me! They carved me up!' I believe I saw tears in my father's eyes too. For the first time since my cutting I had an ally – somebody who was offering sympathy and seemed to be hurting almost as much as I did.

Then my mother rushed in, shouting. 'Leave her alone, Adan! Don't touch her or you'll infect her. It will undo the stitches!'

I have never seen my father so angry. 'How could you?' he raged. 'Why have you done this?'

From the expression on her face, I think my mother was suddenly very ashamed. My grandmother countered that they had only done what was expected of them. I remember she used the expression 'the right thing'. There was a terrible argument between the three of them then in the next room; unlike anything I'd witnessed before. I will always associate it with that day. Listening to their row and seeing how upset my father was by what had happened to me gave me a little courage. It made me realize that this wasn't right. If it had made Father angry then what had been done to me must be wrong.

In silence and with his jaw clenched tightly, he came back into my room with a glass of water, some painkillers, and a few cloths to clean myself with. Grandmother kept telling him not to give me anything to drink, as it would make me urinate before the wound had fused. Tradition prevented him from examining me, sterilizing the cuts or giving me surgical dressings. He remained furious for weeks and continued to support me as best he could from afar, but we both knew it was too late for him to change what had been done.

It was many years before I discovered exactly what the procedure had involved. The old woman, who had the spurious title of 'traditional birth attendant', had sliced off my clitoris and labia minora with her knife and then pared the sides of my labia, removing all the skin right down to the perineum until it was raw and bleeding profusely. Without a surgical glove in sight, she attached the folded edges of my vulva or labia majora to the raw flesh, covering my vagina like a hood. This would eventually fuse together to form a hard bridge of scar tissue that would almost completely restrict the opening. The medical term for it is infibulation, and in what these women considered to be a 'properly infibulated girl' you should not be able to get anything larger than the head of a matchstick into the vagina from that day on until the night of her wedding. This means that whenever urinating or menstruating, urine and blood has to drip-drip out of a hole approximately 1.5–2 mm wide.

I knew nothing of this as a child, of course. I simply lay trapped and isolated in my room, a prisoner of my mother and grand-mother, in agony as the wound began to scab and congeal around the thorns. What hurt the most, though, was the overwhelming sense of betrayal. This changed my relationship with them for ever. Custom dictated that I was to lie on the floor for a week to allow the wound to heal, and hardly drink anything. I was given a little white rice to eat with some sour milk or yoghurt, designed to keep me constipated for several days. But the time came when I needed to empty my bladder, so – although I no longer trusted my mother – I had no choice but to call to her for help. She and my grandmother carried me to the toilet pit and lay me on my side on the floor. 'Go ahead and urinate,' they said, as if it was as simple as that.

Can you imagine? My legs were tied to prevent the wound from opening, I was lying on a dirty and cold cement floor, and the urine wouldn't come. They poured cold water on my feet to make me go, which eventually worked but it stung like crazy. I screamed and tried to halt the flow, but they told me, 'Don't stop. You've got to keep going.'

I didn't believe them so, in what felt like a new form of torture, they kept pouring cold water on my feet to make me start again, and then I longed to empty my bladder completely so that I would never have to endure the pain again. At that point, I also wanted to never drink anything again even though I was so thirsty, because I now knew what fresh agonies a full bladder would bring. Little did I know then that the more concentrated the urine is the more it hurts, so drinking more water would have made it less painful, but nobody told me that.

Just like millions of Somali girls before me and since, I went from one day to the next in my little room, separate from the world and from humanity. Every day, I heard women from the neighbourhood drop in to tell my mother, 'Congratulations, Marian, your daughter has been purified.' What they were purifying an eight-year-old girl from I have no idea. In time, I grew accustomed to turning over gently and to urinating, even though it still hurt horribly. After seven days, the women undid the bindings from my legs and slowly parted them, causing fresh pain. They removed the thorns to see if the wound had fused together, and thank goodness it had – probably thanks to my father's medications. Then they tied my legs together again to keep it from coming undone. They got me to stand up, still bound, and helped me to move about a little one baby step at a time. I felt very dizzy – I had lost a lot of blood and had been lying down for a week. One thing I still remember vividly was the horrible smell of sweat, urine and dried blood that emanated from me, as I hadn't washed for ten days. And this was called purification?

The women who were minding me kept saying, '*Inan baad tahay*, Edna', which means, 'You are a young woman now.' I was no longer an *aruur*, a child. By this they meant that I had been prepared and was ready to be considered for marriage, even though in our culture girls do not generally marry until they are around fifteen (although there are exceptions). As a 'cleansed' virgin, I would be trained to be shy and obedient, respectful and domesticated – the perfect Somali wife.

Eventually the wound mended some more and I was allowed to gently wash myself. They let me sit up, took off my leg bindings and helped me to take a shower. They told me I was healed. Psychologically, I was far from healed. Only then did I understand why the other girls in the neighbourhood had disappeared for three or four weeks and had emerged pale and silent. Just as they must have been, I was terrified that the wound would reopen. Feeling completely alone, I didn't want to see anyone or go out. When I eventually ventured outside, the neighbourhood women constantly reminded me, 'Watch out, don't do too much because if it comes undone we will have to do it again.' You can bet I was careful after that.

Tomboy Edna who'd been such a carefree, rebellious kid had gone for ever. In her place was a frightened little girl who was instructed not to talk about what had happened, which only made me more aloof. While my friends of both genders were playing and singing, laughing and joking, I felt so different. Every time I walked, sneezed or coughed, I remembered the warning that filled me with dread: 'We will have to do it again.'

My grandmother Clara had always been such a comfort and an ally to me, so I longed to see her and have her hold and reassure me, but she was in Borama. By the time she came to visit, my wound had healed and I was already indoctrinated into never speaking about what had happened to me. Later I came to understand that Clara too would have considered my mutilation to be completely normal. From that day on, I regarded all the women in my family with something akin to suspicion, even contempt. They had conspired against me, lied, and disfigured me permanently. How could I ever forgive them?

***

I have never written or spoken about my own experience with female circumcision in any detail before. It isn't easy, but it is time because this mutilating trauma has to stop. Every Somali woman has to live with the memory and then with the physical consequences. It remains with you for life.

Of course the wound heals and gradually you learn to behave normally again. Eventually even the fear that something might happen to undo it subsides. But it takes years to trust people again, or to grow accustomed to the new way of living and urinating. Many teenagers suffer frequent infections and pain. Some even need surgery while menstruating because of blockages, and this has to be done in a certain way and then be certified to prove that the girl's virginity is still intact or she and her family will be dishonoured.

I knew what had been done to me was wrong, but I had no idea what to do about it. Almost every female I knew had gone through the same experience, and virtually everyone younger than me was going to have it done. It took me decades to pluck up the courage to ask questions about the practice, and many more years before I decided to speak out against it.

I wanted to know where and how it started and was astonished to discover that this paganistic ritual pre-dates Islam and Christianity, going back to the fifth century BC and the time of the Pharaohs. In some countries, it is still referred to as 'Pharaonic circumcision'.

The River Nile is the lifeblood of Egypt and the story goes that the god of the river was considered to be the most powerful, and had to be appeased. The most beautiful virgins were chosen for sacrifice and thrown into the river to drown. It was considered an

honour to the family of a girl to be so favoured by the Pharaoh
in order to ensure the survival of her people and the punishment
for refusal was severe. If the river ever dried out or flooded the
fields then it was presumed that the girl chosen hadn't been a
true virgin, which had somehow angered the god. To ensure
that all future 'gifts' would be appropriate, girls were circumcised
and sutured and taken to the temples to be guarded by eunuchs
until it was time for them to be killed. In time, the practice was
adopted as an initiation ceremony by most of the people who lived
along the Blue Nile, which rises in Ethiopia and flows north to
Egypt and the Mediterranean Sea, joining the White Nile from
Burundi. The custom travelled across the equatorial belt through
the Nubian tribe to the Ethiopians, the Sudanese, the Somalis, and
sixteen other countries in Africa as well as a few in Asia. Female
circumcision is largely an accident of geography.

Later, slave traders adopted its use to keep their female 'goods'
from getting pregnant (they also earned more money for virgins),
and nomadic herders also accepted the tradition for population
control or to 'protect' their women from rape. It is still widely
practised by African Muslims, as well as non-Muslims, west of
the Red Sea and the Arabian Sea, as far south as parts of Kenya
and Tanzania. In some instances it is the local blacksmith who
performs the cutting rather than a birth attendant. Nations on
the other side of those two seas don't do it at all, or only so that
it sheds a symbolic drop of blood. In truth, it is not a religious
obligation required by any faith, but primarily a cultural tradition
from a time when people believed in river gods.

Thanks to ignorance and fear, female circumcision is now a
widespread practice that is still carried out on an estimated three
million girls between the age of five and ten every year. In my
country it is estimated that the most severe form, as practised on

me, affects 76 per cent of the female population, a trend that is down from the 100 per cent of my youth and the 98 per cent prevalence we found two decades ago. Because of migration, the practice is also emerging among the refugee communities of Europe and North America, and British hospitals currently treat around 9,000 cases every year.

For now I want to send comforting thoughts to the terrified eight-year-old me who was so bewildered and confused by the heinous thing that was done to her that she still weeps at the cruelty of it.

★★★

When I returned to Djibouti City at the end of that summer I could tell from the look in my Aunt Cecilia's eyes that she knew what had been done to me. Not that she said anything – not even 'sorry'. As I was fast learning, to say nothing about FGM is the considered wisdom among my people.

It was years before I realized that my mother and aunt, as Somali girls from a highly respected family, were also cut but would have been spared the most radical infibulation like mine, and that in French Somaliland Cecilia was free of the social and cultural pressure to have her own daughters 'cleansed'. Rita, Madeleine and Gracie were all untouched, so I was the first daughter of my generation affected. My sister Asha was born in 1948 while I was away at school, and I hoped she would be spared. No such luck.

I now know that families are very often shamed into it, with friends and relatives warning them that their daughters will be spinsters because 'Any husband would expect it.' This is what happened to my mother, who had married young and moved to an environment very different to her childhood. She desperately

wanted to fit in and be seen as a good Muslim wife who'd done
the right thing for me. As the eldest child of Adan Doctor I had
to be of impeccable moral standing.

The pressure to conform doesn't only come from adults.
Children pick up on the language and often tell an 'uncut' girl,
'Keep away from me. Mummy says you still have your shame.
You're not *halal*.' Without even knowing what the procedure
involves, girls beg to be 'cleansed' so that they can be just like
their friends. It is a mystery to them but a natural response from
innocents who also want to fit in. And as in every country where
female circumcision is practised, religion plays no part because it
happens to all girls, be they Christian, Muslim or from a pagan
background. There is little chance of escape.

CHAPTER FOUR

Djibouti City, French Somaliland, 1947

Settling back into my parallel life in a place far from home was all part of the healing process and I embraced my schooling with new fervour. I was there from 1946–1952 and I loved every minute, even though I had the bittersweet knowledge that when I returned to Somaliland my education couldn't be continued.

My brother Farah, who I hardly knew but who joined me at my Aunt Cecilia's when he was eight years old, became my daily companion as we held hands each morning waiting for the school bus. He also embraced our new life in French Somaliland and, in time, we became very close.

We still went back home each summer, spending time with my parents and then holidaying with my grandparents in the country. As soon as school broke up, Farah and I would be driven from Djibouti City to wherever Dad was working, a journey of three or four days. He was usually too busy to pick us up himself, so would send a relative who might also collect other children. For us the journey was the greatest excitement of all, as we passed trees festooned with goats nibbling at the branches, as well as camel herds and donkey caravans in every kind of landscape. One trip home took nine days because of heavy rains. A distant aunt had secured us seats in a truck heavily laden with commercial goods that then became stuck in the mud. There were no phones or other cars on the road to ask for help, so everyone had to help dig it out. Our family knew we were en route but when we didn't show up as expected they were very worried. The only foods we had were onions, salt, tamarind and sweet potatoes, which we roasted. It was on that trip that I learned that peeled bark from an acacia tree could be boiled to make a tea called *asal*. It was cold at night so we drank it to keep warm. Asal is also good for cleaning wounds and sterilizing vessels – a fact I logged for later use.

My brother and I didn't mind being stuck in the middle of nowhere because it felt like a free holiday. The truck was carrying so many interesting people from different tribes all riding on the top, which was heavily laden with goods. My aunt paid extra for us to sleep in the cab at night for safety from wild animals, but Farah and I longed to be up on the roof where our fellow passengers hung off ropes on the sides telling poems and singing songs. There were arguments and running battles, there was love and jealousy and friendship. All of life was there.

Desperate to join them, Farah and I would seek out an old woman or a mother and child and offer them our seats. My aunt praised us for our kindness, never quite appreciating that we did it only so that we could swap places and climb up under the stars to inhale the sweat and the tobacco smoke and listen agog to all the stories.

Life as a child in Africa was such a big adventure.

I always loved reconnecting with my father who'd occasionally take time off to bring us home. I remember him driving us back once and letting me hold the steering wheel while sitting on his lap. Mother was screaming from the back seat, 'Don't let Edna drive, Adan, she'll kill us all!' Dad just laughed and promised to go slowly, letting me steer the car for miles down those bumpy roads and sparking my lifelong love of driving.

Those first summers after my ordeal were when I first started going with him each day to the hospital in Erigavo, the northeastern capital where he was living and working on yet another two-year rotation. I would walk him to the door as I did when I was small but now I'd carry on inside, chattering away and willing to offer my assistance. I was always much happier rolling bandages or washing Dad's medical instruments than peeling potatoes for Mum and – after several catastrophes in the kitchen – she accepted that it was probably better that I didn't help her after all. If we had people coming and I asked if she wanted me to do anything, her answer would be, 'No, no! We have guests today', which told me something about her opinion of my domestic skills. All her life I think Mum believed that my father had gained a daughter in me but that she never really had one. Whenever she told me crossly, 'You're just as bad as your father!' she had no idea that it was the best compliment anyone could pay me.

When Dad came back from work for his meal, I'd be the first to greet him and would occasionally volunteer to make him something he liked. Goodness alone knows what it tasted like, but he always pretended it was delicious and made a big fuss of me. The one thing he especially liked during Ramadan was *labania* – custard made from rice. It was my job to make it – a process that took an entire day, as there was no custard powder back then. First I had to soak grains of fat rice until they expanded, then I had to drain them and scatter them onto a tray to dry in the sun. Then I'd have to pound and sieve it repeatedly until it was powdered, before slowly adding water so as not to make it lumpy. While it was cooking, I'd add cardamom, sugar and milk and then pour it onto little saucers and put them on the windowsill to set, as we had no refrigerator. Dad would taste it, grin and say, 'Hmmm, this is soooo good, Shukri! Only my daughter could have made

this. Did you make it? I knew you did!' He made me feel like
I owned a million camels.

★★★

I was twelve years old during the Year of Red Dust, our country's
worst drought in years, when I became indispensable to my father
at the Erigavo hospital. He not only appreciated my help but also
came to rely on it, especially when the drought and famine gave
him so much extra work.

There are so many more people to deal with in bad times,
and not just those dying of hunger and thirst. Animal carcasses
litter the roads and attract flies that carry more disease. Starvation
compromises the immune system, which gives people a lower
resistance to diseases like TB. Dark hair pales through loss of
pigmentation, skin wrinkles and ankles swell. The children especially suffer from protein calorie malnutrition, also known as
kwashiorkor, or fluid retention in their bellies as their spleens and
livers enlarge. The British-organized military response teams
and the Somali Army set up huge camps in the desert to hold
30–40,000 destitute people. Dad and the Army nursing officers
would travel back and forth to bring the most desperately ill to
the hospital for treatment. Mostly they needed water and food – a
little at a time or they'd die of diarrhoea. We fed them a kind of
gruel or boiled white rice and watered-down milk. If their veins
hadn't collapsed, we could give them saline through a drip. If they
had we were to administer subcutaneous injections daily so that
their bodies could absorb it.

Every morning Dad would ask me to help him with something else. 'Come with me today?' he'd plead. 'There are too
many patients for me to deal with and I need your help with the

dressings.' Or, 'Have breakfast early tomorrow, I want you to assist with a procedure, so dress up and meet me on the ward.' He knew he could trust me that if a surgical instrument needed washing I would do it properly, and that it wouldn't be stolen. We were so short of supplies that the families of patients would be requested to bring in their own sheets, as well as old ones they had no further use for, which I would cut up for dressings. I'd sit in a side room with piles of striped sheets of every colour, ripping and cutting them into every size Dad might need. Every outpatient would also wash their own bandages and bring them back so that we could boil them all up again and issue them with fresh ones. The brand new custom-made bandages from England were kept back for surgery.

My father's single-storey hospital had a male ward, a female ward, a medical ward, a surgical ward, outpatients and a maternity ward. There was room for forty patients. Babies slept with their mothers in their beds as there were no cots and an incubator was unheard of. The staff was largely illiterate and not very conscientious, but the whitewashed building was clean – if a little tired – as it was still inspected by the British once a year.

Dad was run ragged delivering babies, performing minor operations and rehydrating patients. Often he was hampered by the unwritten custom in our country that any surgery or lifesaving procedure on a woman has first to be agreed to by their closest male relative, or the one who is financially responsible for her. Seeking that consent from nomadic families scattered in remote places was often difficult and sometimes impossible to get. He was also much hindered by a lack of supplies, as whatever the British provided was never enough and in times of crisis the demand trebled. He was constantly sending telegrams pleading for extra saline drips or needles, more paraffin, wicks and lamps.

In desperation, he would sometimes put on his best clothes and go in person to see the District Commissioner to ask for what he needed.

I was only permitted to help my father on the outpatient's ward and never near the delivery room. God forbid a Somali girl is let in on the secrets of the female body. If Dad was away visiting the nomads, I was then allowed onto the other wards to supervise those he was most concerned about, help the auxiliaries, and follow the numerous instructions on his list.

My mother objected vociferously. 'Why do you have to go to the hospital again, Edna? What do you know about patients? You'll kill people!'

'I'm not going to kill anybody. I'm just going to make sure the staff are doing what they should be doing.'

'How do you know what they should be doing?'

'I follow what Dad tells me on the piece of paper he left me.'

It never occurred to her to help him, too, or to get some other job. She was a bright, educated woman who'd grown up in a different country, spoke several languages, and could easily have worked as an interpreter or translator. Yet she chose to stay at home to be influenced by her Somali girlfriends about how a wife should be.

★★★

When my schooling in Djibouti City ended after six years, I returned home proudly to Somaliland with my *Certificat d'Études Primaires*. I had done very well, but at fourteen years old I couldn't help but wonder what was in store for me next. Formal education in Djibouti didn't extend beyond primary school, so there was no reason for me to stay and some pressing reasons for me to go home.

Most Somali girls are married between the ages of fifteen and eighteen and if they are still single much beyond that then they are considered not only unmarriageable, but also unlucky. Marriages are often pre-arranged between families, rather than purely for love. Tribal influences are still important and girls are either wed into their own tribe or into a compatible one to establish new alliances. As a naïve teenager, I had no thoughts about marriage and no idea about sex. Anything relating to my private parts was abhorrent to me after my cutting and I couldn't countenance the idea of intimacy of any kind. I enjoyed the weddings of my cousins and other family members with their various ceremonies, dances and feasts, but was puzzled by the notion that Somali men can take up to four wives when I had grown up in an unusually monogamous household.

Instead of boys, my focus was on perfecting my languages. Although I was fluent in French by then, my English was poor – especially my pronunciation – so Dad hired a teacher to show me the correct way to say things by having me study diction and read out loud. Armed with this skill, and with my father's encouragement, I happily jumped at the offer to work for six months as an interpreter for a British doctor named Dr Ashe in the Ruth Fisher Clinic in Hargeisa. This women-only facility had been opened by the Governor's wife in 1945 with an all-female staff designed to encourage Somali women – banned from seeing a male doctor – to attend hospital whenever they were ill or pregnant.

Dr Ashe was an obstetrician married to a fellow doctor and she was very kind to me. I was conscripted into interpreting for her during the morning outpatients' clinic for sick women and children. I didn't know the medical terms for the different medical problems and neither did the patients, but I'd describe their symptoms and the doctor would say, 'Ah, yes, that sounds like cellulitis to me', or, 'I think you may have eczema.' In every case, if she required surgery, each female patient needed to obtain the permission of the male head of her household, which often delayed and complicated treatments, so I had to help with that too. Very often Dr Ashe would be summoned for a difficult delivery so I would also be called. I was usually kept well back but I still witnessed my first births that way, and there was no time to feel squeamish about it. What struck me most of all was how respectful and professional Dr Ashe was and how she worked very hard to keep the mother and baby alive. It was working alongside her that I first learned that the two main killers of pregnant women in my country are poverty and ignorance. A poor nomadic woman who may have started having babies in the bush as a young teenager and could be on her twentieth child by her late thirties has never had any proper medical supervision or social justice. If she starts to bleed out during yet another pregnancy then the chances are that she will die unless her relatives can get her to a hospital.

I was working with Dr Ashe one day when a woman was brought in who'd got into difficulties giving birth at home, which was the first we knew of her – as is often the case. She'd delivered her baby but was haemorrhaging badly and left a sticky trail of blood right into the waiting room. Dr Ashe stayed calm but announced that we had to get her to the operating theatre in Hargeisa Hospital urgently. In spite of transfusions and other measures, this young mother died. Dr Ashe was very upset but still respectful and thanked me for helping her try to save the mother's life. She made me feel important in the equation and she whetted my appetite for even more health work.

When the first boarding school for girls opened almost two hundred kilometres away in the town of Burao in February 1953, Dr Ashe surprised me by recommending to my father that

I be sent there as a pupil teacher. 'Edna shouldn't be wasting her time following me around as an interpreter,' she told him. 'She has the making of something better. She can live in the teachers' accommodation and continue her secondary school education.' There were two British teachers at the Burao school, neither of whom spoke Somali, and one Somali assistant teacher who spoke only limited English. They needed someone with both languages, so I was selected as one of the two pupil-teachers appointed that year. The arrangement was that the staff would give me tutorials after school hours. It was the only option open to me if I wanted to go any further.

For almost two years I lived and worked in Burao, working as an interpreter in the mornings, sitting in on the classes for the first twenty-seven pupils of the new school. I also earned my first wage, which amounted to thirty East African shillings a month plus food and accommodation. I thought I was rich. Every afternoon I had three or four hours of lessons in higher-grade maths, English and biology – all subjects I'd need to pass if I were to one day become a medical assistant to my father. I had to take these lessons alone as it would have been considered improper for me to sit with the high school boys my teacher also taught.

The British authorities had set up a scholarship scheme in which the best students in the Protectorate could be selected to pursue secondary education and professional training in other countries. Scores of teenage boys had already been sent to Aden, Sudan, Kenya and the UK to study anything from engineering to politics, among them several members of my tribe and one from my neighbourhood, Hassan Kayd, who had gone to the prestigious Sandhurst military academy in Britain. Each year a representative from the British Colonial Office came to Somaliland to examine and interview potential candidates for a scholarship, and in 1953, the teachers in Burao put my name on the list – a first for a girl in Somaliland.

The arrival of the British representative, Miss Udell – I'll never forget her name – was a big event in our education system. There was even a countdown to when she'd arrive. It was like a royal visit and the teachers prepared us well with mock exams and staged interviews. First she supervised exams at Sheikh Secondary School and interviewed the boys who obtained top grades, and then she came to Burao to examine a small number of the boys for the scholarship exams – and me. At sixteen years old and approximately five feet tall and weighing fifty kilos, I was the only girl. There was one supervisor for the boys and one supervisor just for me, in a separate room. The Colonial Office must have wondered at Miss Udell's decision to let me sit for the exam and queried whether I would prove a good return to British taxpayers.

To my amazement I passed with flying colours. My father was so proud of me when I told him, but there were problems other than my gender. I was still working towards my secondary school certificate, had a strong French accent, and needed to improve my English. Plus, I was small and skinny for my age, even though I could eat a mountain. Miss Udell considered all these factors and decided that although I'd passed and had good overall grades, I was too young to be sent overseas. 'See you next year, Edna,' she told me with an encouraging smile.

By the time she returned to Somaliland the following year, I had filled out a bit and had one more year of learning and teaching under my belt. I passed the exam once more and could hardly believe it when she told me that I'd won a scholarship to study in England. There were multiple forms to fill in, but when it came to the question that asked me to indicate my preferred course of study, I wrote 'nursing' without a moment's hesitation.

There was one additional hurdle to be overcome before I could be sent to London. The authorities needed to find one other girl to accompany me as a fellow student. The most qualified candidate in the region was Jessica Joseph Raymond from a mission boarding school in Aden who also wanted to be a nurse. Her father was half Indian and her mother half Welsh. Jessica was a delightful young woman; a truly cosmopolitan Somalilander and an ideal companion for someone like me, who'd never travelled further than Djibouti.

CHAPTER FIVE

Jessica and I flew to England in October 1954. I was seventeen years old and she was three months younger. Leaving all that I knew behind, I set off on my big adventure. I'd never been on a plane before so I was agog at our multiple flights in a DC-3 via Aden, Khartoum, Cairo and Athens with eight young Somali men who'd also been selected for a scholarship.

From the moment we arrived at Heathrow airport and were met by representatives from the British Council and the Colonial Office we were treated extremely well. The Somali boys were especially protective of us and anxious that Jessica and I wouldn't be living with them but placed elsewhere. Traditionally, the scholarship boys were put up in a boarding house with older pupils already in the UK who could help them adjust. Jessica and I were such novelties as girls that they didn't know quite what to do with us, so we were put in 'digs'. Our new home was in Balham, south London with a family called the Rodgers. The father worked as a postman and the couple rented out their upper rooms to lodgers. Jessica and I shared one room and there was a tenant in the other. The Rodgers were very welcoming and they introduced us to their children, Gillian, Jacqueline and Roger, who were close to our age and kind to the two strange girls in their midst.

The first thing that struck me about Britain was how cold

and wet it was. I'd read Dickens and the Bronte sisters, so I'd expected rain and autumn mists but not the damp chill. My English vocabulary immediately grew with words like fog and frost, slush and sleet. It also got noticeably darker so much sooner than in Somaliland, where the sun sets and rises roughly the same time all year. We didn't have televisions in Somaliland but we did go to the movies, so we had a general idea of what London looked like. The big city was far larger than I'd imagined, though, with so many cars. What shocked me most were escalators and lifts, neither of which I'd ever seen before and was afraid to use at first.

Perhaps the most memorable initial experience in London was having so much of my own money. The Colonial Office paid us an allowance of £33 a month to cover our rent, breakfast and evening meal, provided by Mrs Rodgers. We could buy lunch at our college and keep the rest of the money back for bus and train fares, and other expenses. They also gave us £50 each with which to buy some clothes suitable for a British winter. Fifty 'quid' was a small fortune and we couldn't believe our luck. A family friend of Jessica's offered to take us shopping, which excited us until he took us to Woolworths and the Army & Navy stores where he insisted that we buy identical shoes, raincoats and hats. We reluctantly did as we were told but kept some money back and the next day went out on our own to the West End.

Oxford Street was like El Dorado to us; we were so amazed by how beautiful and shiny and silky all the clothes were. We blew almost all that was left of our allowance on impractical blouses and silly frilly things that were completely inappropriate. The only scary part of our big day out was taking the Tube. I'd seen trains before in Djibouti but I'd never actually been on one. I didn't know that they could go underground, and that frightened the life out of me, for fear that the roof might collapse or there'd be a flood. To this day, I take the bus rather than the Tube.

Within a few days, I had run out of cash and couldn't afford the train or the bus but I knew I couldn't ask the Rodgers for money. Jessica had an aunt in Cardiff who helped her out, but I had no one, so I went to a post office and sent a telegram to my father.

'*Dear Dad. STOP. Urgently need money for bus fares. STOP. Please send money. STOP. Shukri.*'

The reply came back surprisingly quickly:

'*Don't waste your money sending telegrams. STOP. Make do with what is given to you. STOP.*'

I was so angry with him then. He was a rich man by Somali standards. He was building his own house – as the first Somalilander who'd been allowed to purchase a plot of land in the exclusive European residential area. Yet he was refusing to even send me as much as the sixpenny bus fare to tide me over. I now know that this was exactly the right thing for him to have done and – thanks to Adan Ismail – I have always lived within my means. Embarrassingly, though, I had to borrow money and walk instead of catching the bus until my next month's allowance arrived. That's when I started saving – the best lesson I ever learned from my father.

Because I was not yet eighteen, I couldn't enrol in a nursing programme immediately even if I'd been ready for it, which I wasn't. My scholarship provided for two years of preparatory study that enabled me to complete my secondary schooling and a pre-nursing programme at the Borough Polytechnic in Elephant & Castle, south London. Jessica and I started together at the 'poly' where I was the only black girl in the class (being of mixed race, she was much fairer skinned than I was).

Despite standing out physically, I didn't feel different and quickly made friends. I was popular with the teachers and loved my studies, apart from domestic science in which we had to make hot cross buns and a Sunday roast – things I would never make in Somaliland. If only they'd asked me to make rice custard! As in Djibouti, my biggest challenge was the language. Jessica spoke English far better than I did because she'd done all her basic schooling in it, but once I grasped the language I was away.

There were so few coloured students that I was in demand as a model for the art students to practise pigmentation and skin tones. One of the teachers there also taught in a studio in St John's Wood and paid me £1 per session plus my bus fare to go there one night a week. The students only ever painted my hands, learning how to mix the colours to achieve my particular shade of brown. It may have been unusual for the times, but I don't honestly remember encountering any racism in London. I was more of a curiosity than a threat, like the time I was on the bus and a mother and her young son sat opposite me. The child couldn't take his eyes off my Afro hair and finally asked his mother, 'Can I have a golliwog doll for Christmas?' I didn't say anything but the woman was clearly embarrassed, even more so when I made some response to the ticket collector and the child piped up, 'And can I have one who talks like that?' Seeing the mother's horror, I just smiled and said, 'And I sing too!' as his eyes came out on stalks. I think that put us all at ease.

Later when I was nursing, old ladies seemed especially fascinated by me, but were still always polite. They'd rub my hand with their white sheets to see if the colour came off, or ask questions about life in Africa. One pensioner thanked me for helping her with something before asking, 'Tell me dear, do you people have houses in Africa?' I masked my surprise and told her that, yes, we did. It was a question I was asked very often, and I eventually came up with an answer that tended to prevent further enquiries: 'Why would we have houses when we have trees to hang from?' Perhaps the strangest question of all was, 'Is it true that Africans have a tail?' I was so taken aback that I replied, 'Yes, but I had mine cut off.' Seeing a Nigerian nurse working on the other side of the ward, I suggested, 'Why don't you ask if she still has hers?'

Aside from the Rodgers family, Jessica and I were also under the benign supervision of a guardian from the Colonial Office, Colonel William Vernon Crook, who'd recently retired from his position as Director of the Department for East Africa and Aden affairs. The colonel, who had a daughter our age and an unmarried sister called Mouse, took Jessica and me under his wing. He had a cottage on the Thames where he kept a boat, so he and his family would take us on cruises up the river and to Kew Gardens to see the tropical plants. He introduced us to horticulture and took us to the Chelsea Flower Show, an annual event attended by the Queen that we'd never otherwise have known about or made time for. I don't know if the colonel's prize-winning roses ever made it to Chelsea, but that kind old man with the handlebar moustache gave me a lifelong love of growing plants.

Around this time, I found myself some part-time work reporting on life in the UK for the BBC, which had a relay station in Berbera that broadcast a daily Somali programme of news and events across East Africa. The 'Beeb' constantly required new material and would store future fillers, it's not like milk that can go bad. Somebody at a party asked me if I'd like to contribute, as they wanted female voices for a female audience. I told them I didn't know how but they sent me to a woman who taught me how to speak slowly into a microphone, take the right number of breaths and never rustle my papers. An engineer and an editor guided me and my reviews about British cultural events were never live so they could always edit out my many mistakes.

To my delight, I was given tickets for the Ideal Home exhibition at Olympia, the ballet at Sadler's Wells, and concerts at the Royal Festival Hall, reporting on them to my people. I also provided the female voices for some of their regular entertainment programmes such as *1001 Nights*. One of my fellow reviewers was a Somali Army cadet called Abdullahi Said Abby, a charming young man who was training in London and who I frequently bumped into at receptions. The BBC paid me five guineas if I was working from a script written for me, and extra if I wrote the script myself. That was a lot of money for a student in those days. If I recorded two or three programmes at once, I'd take home fifteen guineas when a student nurse would only earn eight guineas a month. Working for the BBC helped pay for driving lessons (something I wouldn't have been allowed to do back home), and enabled me go on holidays to Amsterdam, Paris and the Austrian Tyrol with friends.

The biggest thrill about my work for the BBC was that my father heard me on the radio, and wrote immediately to express his surprise and pride. 'How do you find the time in between your studies?' he asked. My mother, who only ever signed the bottom of his many letters to me with, '*Love from Mum*', didn't make any comment.

★★★

The departments and classes at Borough Polytechnic were enormous and I had to adjust to being surrounded by hundreds of teenagers also studying for their O levels in everything from pre-dentistry or pre-medicine to engineering and catering. Those two years were a great experience and forced me to develop better study habits. During my time there I prepared for the state preliminary examination for nursing and also did the equivalent of the first term of Nursing School. This exempted me from one semester of the nursing programme once I was admitted.

One day a week we were taken for some practical experience to the Victorian Belgrave Hospital for Children near the Oval cricket ground in Kennington, south London. In huge, efficient wards, unrecognizable to me from anything I'd experienced in Somaliland, I worked alongside nurses, washed babies, fed and changed them, read to the older children, and helped give them their medication. It was our job to get the more mobile patients out of bed and take them to the window or wrought iron balcony for some fresh air. It was basic, uncomplicated care and we were given no responsibility in case we did something dangerous. I'd done much more practical nursing at home for my dad and was itching to get on, but I wasn't old enough or good enough yet.

My early years in London weren't all about work, though – far from it – and Jessica and I could be quite mischievous at times. On the last Saturday of every month there were college dances known as 'hops'. As this was the Fifties the music was largely swing and jazz featuring singers like Doris Day, Rosemary Clooney, Perry Como, Frank Sinatra and Dean Martin. Although I'd listened to my mother's records when I was small, it was in London that I really discovered music for the first time. I bought my first record player, a secondhand Grundig, and spent ages browsing through the Ella Fitzgerald and Louis Armstrong albums in record shops. I even queued to see Harry Belafonte perform at the Hammersmith Palais. A few of us also learned to dance so that we could show off at the hops. From then on, dancing became my number one hobby. With my pinched-in, 22-inch waist accentuated by a flared tulle underskirt and my Afro tamed into the tight chignon, I learned the tango, the quickstep, the foxtrot and the rumba.

The music department provided the musicians for these events and the catering students made the food and sold the drinks, so the whole college was involved. Dancing is thirsty work and one night Jessica and I spent so much on orange squash that we didn't have the Tube fare home. We began to walk, but had no idea of the direction. The Rodgers had told us that if we ever had a problem we should find a policeman, so we walked and walked looking for a 'bobby' until we found two on foot patrol. We always carried a piece of paper with our address in it – 137 Ramsden Road – so we showed it to them and explained that we were lost.

'Goodness, you're a long way from home!' one of the officers exclaimed. 'Just a moment.' He went to a telephone box, called up his police station and before we knew it a squad car arrived to pick up two 'lost' girls – who weren't lost at all really – and drove us all the way to Balham. We arrived at about 1 a.m. and a policeman rang on the doorbell (waking the whole household) and handed us over to the Rodgers, telling them, 'We found these two waifs.' Mr Rodgers thanked them for their kindness and we all went to bed. Very cheekily after that we made one more attempt to use the Metropolitan Police as a kind of personal taxi service. We even made a game of it, walking miles in the search for different policeman to trick into taking us home. In the end, word got around and the long-suffering officers told us, 'No more!'

After my first Christmas in London, I attended a New Year's Eve ball for overseas students and their host families arranged by the British Council. This gala event had a big band and lots of dancing. I don't recall the venue, but I do recall the handsome man who came up to ask me for a dance. While we were waltzing, he asked, 'Where are you from?'

'Somaliland,' I replied.

He stopped dancing and stared at me.

I laughed. 'What, don't you know where Somaliland is?'

He shook his head in disbelief. 'Yes, I do. I am from Somaliland too!'

It was my turn to be shocked. 'No! Then w-who are you?' I stammered. I thought I knew all the students from Somaliland, but here was a Somali I'd never encountered.

'Well, who are you?' he countered.

'I am Edna Adan Ismail,' I told him, knowing that the mention of my father's name never failed to impress someone from my country. It worked. He couldn't believe it and said that he was directly related to my mother. His name was Mohamed, the twenty-six-year-old son of Haji Ibrahim Egal, whose family I knew. I spent the entire evening dancing with him after that and when we parted I gave him my address and phone number.

The next day the first bouquet I ever received in my life was delivered to Ramsden Road. The enormous cluster of roses from a handsome older man made quite an impression on a naïve seventeen-year-old. I kept the note I found nestling in among the blooms for many years. It said:

'Thank you for such a wonderful, delightful evening. Do you realize that we made history – probably the first Somalis who danced together in England? Mohamed.'

Mrs Rodgers found a vase to put my flowers in, and for several weeks they brightened up the living room we shared. I was not a very romantic person and had never been out with any boy before, unless in a group. I was too passionate about my work to have time for romance and anyway the Somali tradition was that you never 'messed around' until you got married. Not that I could – my circumcision made that decision easy – and any boy who violated the daughter of Adan Dhakhtar Ismail and robbed me of my virginity would be considered to have raped me, with terrible repercussions for his family. There would have been vendettas and rebellions, as this was one code of ethics you did not break.

Nevertheless, a few days later Mohamed invited me to dinner and I accepted. To my surprise, he arrived in a convertible sports car. This was the first inkling I had of his fondness for expensive, showy things; but then I remembered that his father was reportedly one of the richest men in Somaliland. All the neighbours peered out of their windows and I could almost see their blinds twitching as I climbed into the red MG. We had a lovely evening and he took me to dinner a couple of times after that, but then he simply disappeared. I never heard a word from him. Mrs Rodgers would ask, 'Whatever became of that nice young man who sent you flowers?' I had no answer, because I didn't know what had happened to him. We hadn't fought, we hadn't argued. He just vanished. It was almost a year later when I learned that his father had suffered a stroke and he'd flown back to Somaliland in a hurry. As the only surviving child of a mother who'd been pregnant eighteen times and lost her other son to a snakebite, Mohamed's duty was to be by her side. Haji Ibrahim Egal died six months later, and Mohamed remained to run the family business, forgetting to write to a girl he'd once sent flowers to in London.

After a year with the Rodgers, Jessica and I bade them a fond farewell and moved into a boarding house run by nuns at 24 The Boltons, off the Old Brompton Road in Kensington. It was a place that took in mainly rich girls from abroad studying the arts. The property was a fine white stucco building with individual bedrooms and a common dining room. It was located in a very fashionable part of town, closer to the station and with a more frequent bus service. We loved living there and when we weren't working, we went to the movies or to dances with friends. I recall that one of the films I saw that I enjoyed the most was called *The World of Suzie Wong*, starring the Hollywood heartthrob William Holden. Once a week we'd have social evenings where we were each invited to discuss our cultures. Jessica and I learned all about Ireland, the Gambia, China, India, Portugal and Finland from the other girls before it was our turn to don traditional Somali nomad dress – six metres of unstitched white cloth tied a bit like a sari and adorned with amber beads – and sing Somali songs. It was a great way to break the ice.

It was a lot of fun living in the centre of cosmopolitan London. I was made so welcome and enjoyed my newfound freedom. Despite the parties and the pranks, however, I remained a diligent student and passed all my exams – including anatomy and physiology – with good grades. I did so well, in fact, that my teachers hinted that I might consider switching from nursing to medicine, but I was undecided about that and resolved to ask my father's advice when I was next back home. The previous few years had brought about such momentous changes, yet there I was, eighteen years old, living in a very different kind of world and with my nursing studies about to begin. I was no longer a frightened little girl, confused by life's mysteries and holding onto my father's hand. I was a young woman doing as I pleased, on the brink of my chosen career. Life was good.

★★★

In the summer of 1956, I went home for the first time in two years. This was something that had always been promised by the Colonial Office and was much anticipated by those of us who'd been away so long.

Everything seemed smaller than I remembered but it was good to be back. I'd been especially homesick for spicy curries and chilli peppers. The food in London seemed so bland by comparison to our Indian-influenced cooking. I had also missed my brother Farah and my younger sister Asha, then eight. I wished my grandmother Clara were still alive so I could go to Borama with her and drink cow's milk, but the herd had been sold long ago and she'd died of cancer of the uterus before I left for Britain. Most of all, I wanted to see my dad. By then he'd finished building his house – one of the first in Hargeisa to have electricity and a telephone (connected to an exchange) – and he even owned his own car. For the first time in his working life he was no longer dependent on the British government for accommodation or transport. My parents were proud of me, or at least my father was. Mum never said much and I'm sure she wanted me to give up my dream, come home and settle down. Her most oft-repeated comment was, 'I married a crazy husband and he gave me a crazy daughter.'

I was delighted to learn that my cousin Gracie from Djibouti would be spending the summer with us. She was only eight months younger than me and we'd been close at school, so I loved reconnecting and catching up on all the news of Aunt Cecilia and the rest of the family. Having had unlimited freedom in Britain, I was even more independent than before, so Gracie and I went out on our own, as carefree and unescorted as if we were living in London or Djibouti. I was careful not to upset my mother and knew my behaviour would raise eyebrows among her friends and family, but I also knew how important it was to remain true to who I was. In fact, I was hardly ever at home because of all the invitations I received, many of them from the British because of my father's status, but also because the authorities wanted to be reassured that they hadn't wasted their money sending me abroad.

They were relieved to find a young woman who dressed like them and spoke their language, and pleased to know that I was doing well.

The reaction from the Somali women couldn't have been less encouraging, however. Everyone voiced their opinion and my mother's cousins, neighbours, friends and aunts continually reminded me that as a woman I didn't need to learn how to be anything. The rest of my family was chiefly focused on the honour of the tribe and were quick to warn me I was jeopardizing myself and the rest of the clan. 'If you carry on working and living like a Westerner, you will never be considered worthy of marriage,' I was informed. 'This will reflect badly on the women in our family, especially your mother who'll be harshly judged for having brought you up unprepared for a life of marriage and domesticity.'

I was so committed to my studies by then that nothing anyone could say would put me off. As far as I was concerned, my only decision was to choose between nursing and medicine. This dilemma arose after the completion of my first year of pre-nursing training when Colonel Crook called me in for a chat. After closely studying copies of all of my grades and supervisors' reports, he told me, 'Look, Edna, you are getting good grades, your teachers respect you, and everyone is very happy with your progress. Given your performance, you might want to know that we would consider changing your scholarship from nursing to medicine.'

Goodness, I was only a teenager and my brain was still growing. I seriously considered his offer but told myself, 'Medicine? That will take me six or seven more years. My God, I'll be so old when I finish! It is too long. I'm going to stick to nursing.'

Colonel Crook advised me to think about it and I suspect he hoped that I'd discuss it with my father when I went home. My instinct told me that Dad would say: 'Medicine, of course', and

I didn't want that pressure on me, so in the end I didn't even ask him. When I got back to London, Colonel Crook asked, 'What's it going to be then, nursing or medicine?'

'Nursing,' I replied decisively.

'Are you sure? Have you discussed this with your family?'

'I don't need to discuss this with anyone. This is my life and it is my decision. This is what I want to do.'

CHAPTER SIX

London, England, 1956

The happiest years of my youth were spent as a student nurse. From as far back as I could remember I'd dreamed of putting on a uniform and a peaked cap and becoming the efficient, medically trained assistant that Dad so desperately needed, in a hospital that was worthy of him. The first part of my dream was finally coming true.

When it was time to apply to nursing school, I chose the West London Hospital in Hammersmith and was accepted for a three-year course, coupled with a variety of rotations throughout London and the Home Counties. I moved out of The Boltons and into the far less salubrious Abercorn Nurses' Home in Hammersmith Road, a building that had first been opened at the end of the First World War. I had been waiting so long to start my studies that I felt ready for anything. I knew that the training would be hard and understood that it would take many years for me to make it to senior sister, but that was what I wanted more than anything in the world. I am, by nature, a hoarder and I especially like to hoard knowledge. All my life I have soaked up new information, new words, new experiences, and this – I was confident – was going to be one of the greatest experiences of all.

One thing I hadn't expected was that before I even started the course I was required to have a medical examination. Part of this involved providing a urine sample. When the results returned, it showed that I had an abnormally high white blood cell count that could be a sign of infection or contamination. To be certain that I wasn't suffering from kidney disease, they demanded that a specimen of urine be collected via a sterile catheter. Panicking, and knowing that because of my infibulation I couldn't possibly give such a sample in the normal way, I refused. The Sister in charge immediately assumed that I had a sexually transmitted disease or some other infection and brusquely told me, 'If you can't have the medical, you can't go into nursing.'

Mortified, I didn't know what to do. I had never spoken to a soul about my cutting and wasn't even aware then that other women went through it, too. Because of it, I was one urine sample away from being rejected for the course I had waited all my life for – the first time that I had been faced with any consequences. Seeing how upset I was, a junior Sister kindly took me to one side and asked, 'Tell me the truth, Edna. Do you have an infection?'

Wiping away my tears, I shook my head.

'Are you refusing the catheter because you have an obstruction?' she enquired, gently.

I looked up, shocked. How did she know? I could only think that she must have come across the problem before.

I nodded.

She patted my hand reassuringly and said, 'I won't ask you to show me. I will take your word for it.' Somehow, she arranged that my medical examination could continue with a mid-stream specimen of urine, an X-Ray and blood sample instead, for which I was eternally grateful. I didn't know it then but have since learned that because of the skin covering the urethra in girls who've been cut, urine bounces against the artificial wall back into the

vagina, flushing out dead cells. This means that it often contains
more white cells, which can be indicative of an infection. This
stagnation of menstrual flow, urine and normal secretions causes
infections to spread and can interfere with fertility. Thankfully,
my medical examination was clear and I was allowed to continue
my nursing training.

Once I was enlisted, my name created my next problem because
I was incorrectly listed as Nurse Adan instead of Nurse Ismail,
which meant that I was paired with Nurse Adams, who was horribly accident-prone. After I had them correct the administrative
error, I was paired instead with Nurse Harrison, the brightest
student of us all. By competing with someone of her talent I had
to work extra hard, but it was she as much as anyone who pushed
me to excel.

Not that it was all plain sailing. Like all rookies, I made my fair
share of mistakes, especially when it came to understanding the
nuances of the English language. To begin with I was on a six-
week rotation between departments to get a flavour of everything
from orthopaedics to outpatients. During my first few days on a
surgical ward my supervisor asked me to 'special' a man who'd
just had his appendix removed and was coming round from the
anaesthesia. This was the term used to give a patient special care.

The curtains were drawn around his bed and when I approached
and peered inside, I could see that he was very woozy and diso-
rientated. In those days, surgical patients were given a lot of
chloroform and ether that often made them sick and agitated. This
was my first semi-conscious case and I was extremely nervous.
The man looked up, saw me and, in a strong Cockney accent,
asked, 'Oh, Nurse, me innards! What have you done with me
innards?' I had no idea what he was talking about and certainly
didn't know what 'innards' meant. I presumed that it must be

something valuable such as a wedding ring, spectacles or maybe his dentures – the kind of things that patients are always looking for – so I tried to reassure him that his innards were safe and started looking around to see where they might be. There was nothing obvious on his bed or bedside table, so I opened his locker to see if I could find what he wanted inside. Just at that moment the supervisor returned, saw me rummaging around in a delirious patient's personal belongings, and asked, 'What on earth are you doing, Nurse?'

'I'm looking for his innards, Sister,' I replied in all seriousness. 'The patient is most concerned about them, so I wanted to find them for him.' The look on her face was one I shall never forget. From that day on I became known to all on that ward not as Nurse Ismail or Nurse Somali, but as 'Nurse Innards'. It took me a long time to live that one down.

On another occasion, a patient asked me to fetch him the caviar that a friend had brought in for him, which had been placed in the staffroom fridge. I had no idea what caviar was and went to look for it, but found nothing. I reported back that it wasn't there whereupon he created quite a scene. It was only later that I realized that the stinky black mess I'd thrown out of the fridge earlier that morning for being off was the eye-wateringly expensive Beluga that everyone was now looking for.

My most frightening case happened when I was on a night shift on the top floor surgical wing of the West London. It was a ward of about twenty beds and I sat at the nurse's table at the far end with an angle poise lamp bent low over my books so as not to disturb the patients. One of them had recently had a prostatectomy and was in a bed nearest the window. The drain in his bladder had metal clips that banged against the bottle or the side of his bed, making a clanking sound whenever he moved. I was still working on my assignment when I heard the familiar clank and suspected he was turning over. I lifted my light towards him to check and couldn't immediately see anything untoward, but turned it higher to give him one last look.

To my horror I saw that he had crept out of bed, pushed up the sash window and had one foot over the windowsill as if to jump. Running as fast as I could, I grabbed his foot, but he was a big man and I knew I'd never hold onto him. Shrieking, I cried out for help and another patient jumped out of bed and helped me pull him back inside. The delirious jumper kept saying, 'I won't be gone long, Nurse. I'll be back in a minute.' He had no idea he was on the top floor and would have died. Plus, I would have been shot at dawn. Luckily, life as a student nurse wasn't always so troublesome and on the whole was exciting and fun. I fully embraced the experience of every new department I went to, making private mental notes if I found some aspect of it that I admired – such as an efficient sterilization system – or of which I disapproved – such as poor lighting or an inferior layout. I was determined that the hospital that I built one day for my father would have only the best.

I next applied to take a short rotation in an STD clinic for sexually transmitted diseases. This was something Dad had studied, and that was extremely relevant in Somaliland, where he frequently treated people for gonorrhoea and syphilis. I had a remarkable Principal Tutor at West London called Miss Markham, who became one of my mentors. When I asked her for the STD rotation, however, she looked at me curiously and asked me why. Most people wouldn't volunteer for such an experience and I think she must have wondered if I had an STD. 'I need to know how to take care of these kinds of patients back home,' I told her quickly. 'My father treats people for gonorrhoea and syphilis quite often.'

I was still young, but I had to think ahead and imagine what I'd be dealing with once I started working at his side. Miss Markham understood and granted me my wish.

The busy STD clinic was open from early in the morning until very late at night. The patients each had a number; we never knew their identities or saw their names, so it was all very discreet and anonymous. People would come in for their penicillin or other injections in their own cubicle, to give them privacy so they didn't see each other or people they knew. Often they'd drop in before work or afterwards. In those days there was no AIDS yet, thank God, but there were genital ulcers and all manner of other nasty problems. You would never have guessed that these smart, elegant people in suits and dresses with busy working lives had the most distressing diseases. I knew very little about homosexuality or men courting men when I arrived at that clinic but I soon learned and it was a real eye-opener.

The STD rotation was a great experience for me and another test of my resilience. It was two weeks of remarkable efficiency and discretion, which proved invaluable in later years. I learned so much in the STD clinic, not least that I had to be meticulous in sterilizing the instruments and always wear my gloves and mask as I didn't want to catch anything or give it to someone else.

My first rotation away from the West London after I'd earned my second-year stripe was to spend three months at St Mark's Hospital in the City, which specialized in diseases of the rectum and colon. There I learned about everything from colostomies to haemorrhoids, in patients young and old. Then in my third year I was sent to Clare Hall Hospital in South Mimms, Hertfordshire, where my father had also trained. This depressing place, with approximately five hundred patients in what felt like the middle of nowhere, was my least favourite placing as a nurse. An isolation hospital first opened in the 1800s by a charity to treat smallpox in the poor, Clare Hall became a specialist centre for TB and terminal lung cancer patients.

TB is a big problem in developing countries, aggravated by AIDS these days. Many patients who have a compromised immune system catch TB, which is described as 'an opportunistic disease'. The death rate in the 1950s was exceptionally high – around forty per cent. Treatment was a long, tedious business in which patients had to spend at least eighteen months in a sanatorium. It was thought they needed fresh air, so they were placed in open-sided post-war EMS huts or emergency medical shelters and even slept there (wrapped in blankets) during the winter. There was little proof that it helped, but nobody really knew and it seemed to make sense.

Every nurse had to be vaccinated and wear a mask at all times before being allowed to work in this large, forbidding building which felt like something out of a Dickens novel. It had huge grounds with trees and lakes surrounded by buildings for different categories of patients, each located according to their state of recovery. The most highly infectious were placed some distance from the others, and the ones almost ready to go home were given tasks to keep them busy such as wheeling library books around, helping the nurses roll gauze pads, or making cotton wool balls for injections.

Every Sunday we had to clean the wards, which meant scrubbing the floors and swabbing down the walls. Each patient had their own thermometer kept in a test tube dipped in alcohol and hung above their bed. My assignment one day was to wash and sterilize all the thermometers and put them back in new test tubes with fresh alcohol. Simple. I collected them up and ran warm water over them in the basin as I'd been trained, but then a fellow student came in and started talking to me. Distracted, I kept the tap running too long until it became scalding hot and popped the lot. Mortified, I laid them on a tray and took them to the Sister to tell her what had happened.

'Well, how many did you break?' she asked.

'All sixteen.'

'What? How did you do that? Nobody has ever broken sixteen thermometers before! Don't you know that hot water breaks thermometers, Nurse?'

'Yes, Sister, but I wasn't paying attention. It was an accident. I'm sorry.' She wouldn't let the matter go and insisted that she couldn't have those kinds of accidents on her ward. I should have just kept apologizing but instead I offered to pay for replacements out of my own money, which made her see red.

'How dare you! You think if you make a mistake you can simply fix it with money? What if you make a mistake with a life, or a dosage? How will you pay for that?' She declared that she would no longer have me on her ward and sent me to my overall boss, the Matron, to be reassigned. Terrified that this might be the end of my career, I hurried to my room to change into a freshly starched apron (you never went to see Matron with a dirty apron) and prepared to admit my mistake. She was warned that I was on my way and I walked like a condemned prisoner through the hospital towards her office feeling that everyone from the porter to the secretary was looking at me as if I was a monster. 'There goes the girl who broke sixteen thermometers!' I imagined them saying. In the history of Clare Hall nobody had ever committed such a crime.

Matron gave me a good dressing down in what proved to be my first and last warning. My day off was cancelled; I had to pay for my mistake in time and money, and was warned to be more careful in the future. From that day on I picked up thermometers as if they were butterflies that might crumble in my fingers. Even today I tell my students to watch out, as they are far more difficult to replace in Somaliland.

★★★

The majority of our patients at Clare Hall were men, many of whom had served in the war. They came from all classes and most had been heavy smokers, as was the norm. We often had to confiscate cigarettes and matches brought in by relatives. Those dying of lung cancer knew they had no chance of survival, as there was no radiotherapy or chemotherapy and only palliative care. We all knew what would happen to them, which made caring for them all the more depressing.

The worst part of being at Clare Hall, however, was the treatment we had to administer to the TB patients, many of whom caught the bacillus at a time when vaccinations weren't that common. Most needed to be given a handful of pills every day as well as daily painful intramuscular injections of streptomycin antibiotic into their buttocks. These men were emaciated with hardly any flesh and our overused and repeatedly boiled and blunted needles would often hit their hipbones and cause them to cry out in pain. Abscesses would develop on the injection sites, making the next jab worse. I hated that assignment more than any other, but it couldn't be avoided. After months of such treatment the men often became depressed and hopeless. However hard I tried to lift their spirits by chattering away cheerfully they wouldn't respond. As if that wasn't bleak enough, the hospital – which was rumoured to be haunted by the 'grey lady' ghost of a lovesick nun who drowned herself in the pond – was miles from anywhere and almost impossible to take a break from. Transport to and from London involved walking along a dark lane between fields before a convoluted journey by bus and Tube. There were always cattle or horses snorting and puffing on the other side of the high hedges, especially on the return journey at night, which was especially scary for a girl from Africa where any animal is potentially lethal.

All of the nurses were accommodated in a residential block where, for some reason, I was the only one assigned a room on the ground floor alongside the senior staff nurses and sisters. My window opened onto a pleasant lawn. As soon as the rooms were allocated, I found that I was very popular. 'We have a room on the ground floor!' one of my fellow students cried.

'We?' I said. 'What's this *we*? It's a small single room and I'm not sharing with anybody.' They explained that there was a standing rule that anybody with a room on the ground floor had to agree to the others gaining access after curfew as the front door was locked at midnight. As I hardly ever left the building, this proved to be a nuisance as my friends were frequently climbing in and out. After a few weeks of this, I made the stipulation that they all come home at the same time so that I wasn't repeatedly awoken. I also moved my bed from directly beneath the window so that they wouldn't tread on me. Night after night, they'd creep in with a whispered, 'Thank you, Edna', before slipping upstairs.

One night they asked me to join them. We had a wonderful evening with dinner and a movie at the Odeon Leicester Square before catching the Tube to High Barnet for the long journey back through the fields, giggling all the way. We arrived back at the hospital past midnight but I'd left my window unlocked. The problem was that I didn't immediately recognize which was my window because I'd never had to before. As one window was open, though, I assumed it to be the one and was the first to climb in. The girls helped me up but when my foot came into contact with a bed I knew immediately that this couldn't be my room after all. Before I could retreat, I heard a woman cry out, 'What? Who's that? Thief! Thief! Rapist! Rapist! Help me! Help!!' A firm hand grabbed my ankle and wouldn't let go, no matter how much I resisted. As I struggled, the girls outside thought that I was about to fall so they pushed me further in, whereupon I realized that it was one of the sisters who was screaming and crying. Somehow I managed to extricate myself from her grip and tumble back out. Before all hell broke loose, we hurried along to the right window, lifted the sash and clambered in like sheep jumping over a fence.

As the girls fled upstairs before the lights came on, the sister next door was still screaming about a rapist. Fully clothed, I slid under my sheets and pretended to be asleep. The Night Sister came around banging on all the doors and asking, 'Are you okay, Nurse? Lock your doors and windows. There's a rapist about.' When the security guards came to my room to check on us all, I was still buried under my blankets. 'Put out the lights, please,' I muttered. 'I'm trying to sleep.'

The following morning the news had gone all around the hospital. A 'big rapist with huge muscles' tried to rape the sister who bravely fought him off. The girls and I had to suppress our smiles. The muscly arm she claimed to have battled with was actually my ankle, which was as thin as a roll of gauze. Needless to say, that night marked the end of anyone using my window again, much to everyone's disappointment.

One of my fellow students, Nurse Adams (the clumsy one I was first paired with), had a far worse experience at Clare Hall. Every morning we'd give the men a cup, a bowl and some hot water so that they could wash themselves and shave. We'd draw their curtains around them to do their ablutions in private and then ask if they'd finished so that we could take everything away. One of Adams' patients, a terminally ill man in his forties, didn't respond so she pulled back the curtain to check if he was finished. To her horror, she saw that he had slashed his wrists with his razor blade and was bleeding into the washbowl. When she screamed, he told her, 'Stay where you are Nurse! Don't come near me!' As she rushed forward to grab the razor, he slit his own throat.

The few patients who were mobile jumped out of their beds and ran to help her. They got the razor out of his hand so that his wounds could be tended to. Adams bound his wrists and tried to stop the bleeding, but he'd lost so much blood that it was too late. He'd had enough. By the time the police arrived he was dead and she was in shock. This only added to my grim Clare Hall experience and I was so pleased when my three months was up. I wrote and asked my father about his time there and he said he'd had very different experiences, none of which had been bad at all. It took me a lot of nursing years to appreciate that doctors don't see things the same way nurses do. They don't experience the reality. They go on their rounds and ask a few questions and only see the medical side. 'What's his blood count now? What did the lab results say? Okay, then do this or prescribe that.' Then they go on their way.

We nurses are on the front line and see the patients every day. We register their moods, depressions and small setbacks or improvements. We know if they are sad or worried. We see how differently they behave when relatives come and they try to put on a brave front. As a nurse you can't help but get involved with the emotional part of your patients' lives. You become so immersed in their daily troubles that you develop almost a silent conspiracy against the doctors. The emotional side of things is so important and if you cannot deal with it, then nursing isn't a job for you. At Clare Hall, I learned that if you don't have the compassion or the human touch, then you will never be a good nurse.

★★★

The rotation I enjoyed best of all was in surgery. I think what appealed to me most was the efficiency. Working in an operating theatre was fast and clean and everything took place in an extremely decisive atmosphere. There was a beginning, middle and an end. You found the problem, cut it out, fixed it, closed up and sent the patient back to the ward. There was such a satisfying sense of accomplishment, unlike anything I had experienced before.

The senior nurse in charge of the entire surgical complex at West London was a woman named Theresa Monk, who signed herself 'T. Monk', so the student nurses gave her the nickname 'Tiger Monk'. She became my hero, even though she never, ever got my name right. She ran those theatres like a ship. In her early fifties, she was agile, knowledgeable, and authoritative. She anticipated the needs of the surgeons (who were also afraid of her) and was on top of everything. She was also so demanding and unforgiving that student nurses said that being assigned to work under her was like serving a prison sentence. The equipment had to be just right, the instruments perfectly sterile, and the patient properly prepared. Many a girl had sleepless nights ahead of their surgical rotation and some were so nervous in her presence that they made terrible mistakes.

I didn't find her intimidating at all. To my mind she was the best supervisor I had ever worked for and a most powerful female role model. Aside from Aunt Cecilia, it was the first time I'd seen that in a working woman. Tiger Monk was so capably in command of her department that had life and death in its hands. She never raised her voice, but you knew when she disapproved, and she kept her entire team on its toes. 'How dare you put that dirty instrument here, Nurse,' she'd say, as her eyes bored into a hapless junior. 'Couldn't you have opened those forceps and scrubbed in between? Don't you know how much of a risk that is to a patient? If that's how you want to run things then you can go and work in a butcher's shop. We're paid to save lives not kill patients.'

My father adopted a far gentler way of training his staff, but there was something of him in her that I admired enormously. There was only one way to do things and that was her way, the proper way. Whatever she told me to do, I did to the best of my ability. I wasn't afraid of her and looked forward to working with her so that I could learn something. Perhaps because of this, I soon became the teacher's pet. Tiger Monk would allow me to scrub and assist her and when she saw that I had the hang of it, she'd remove her gloves and say, 'You are doing quite well, Nurse, carry on.' I'd be left to hand the surgeon his instruments, while she flitted around and kept an eye on me from a distance. That is how I was trained and how I came to love the operating theatre.

From then on, I always watched for new postings on the surgical schedule. If there was an emergency aortic aneurysm, even if it was on my day off, I'd beg to be allowed to attend because I knew this wasn't something I could see every day. There were very few students who'd forfeit their one day off a week to watch an operation. I think my enthusiasm endeared me to Sister Monk because she began to tell me if there was an upcoming splenectomy, nephrectomy (the removal of a kidney), or a brain tumour operation and give me the chance to assist. She showed confidence in me and she trusted me, which boosted my morale enormously.

Best of all, I became part of the operating team. When the head nurse needed something – 'Go and find me a number 1 catgut' – I knew where to find it. If she dropped an instrument, I would fetch her a clean one. I assisted at minor operations such as tonsillectomies, appendectomies and hernias and watched in awe as the table was set up by professionals based on a precise diagram of where each instrument should be placed. I learned that if you focused on your work and enjoyed it as much as I did, there really was no way for you to go wrong.

I still miss the silence and precision of the operating theatre. The atmosphere is like no other. There is no tension, just professionalism. What these surgeons did was such a miracle of medicine that I was in awe. It is then that I was most tempted to switch to medicine but Tiger Monk taught me enough. She shaped me professionally, and thanks to her I won a second prize in surgical nursing (after Nurse Harrison, of course). I resolved to make sure that I had a Tiger Monk in my hospital and, oh boy, what my father would have given for one like her in Somaliland!

Of course not every operation goes well and there are some patients who can't be saved. Even those who wake up from the anaesthesia don't really know what went on in the theatre, or how close they came to dying. As a nurse, you follow them through the post-operative recovery and, if all goes well, you watch them go home. Sometimes they get an infection, have a heart attack or something goes wrong and they are dead before you can even run to the telephone. I was on a medical ward at the West London when I had to deal with my first body. I'd only ever seen a dead pet and my baby brother, but I was too young then to make much sense of it. I knew that patients died in my father's hospital, but I wasn't allowed onto the wards unless I'd been sent by someone to look for him. Only then might I wander in and know someone was close to death because of the numbers of family members around the bed, but I'd always be shooed out before I saw anything too unpleasant. Even when that mother bled out, I was ushered away before the end.

Now it was very different. When a patient died in our care, there were rituals we had to perform. Supervised by a senior or staff nurse, we washed the deceased in pairs and helped plug all the orifices. We wrapped them in a shroud and made sure that they were left in a position that was dignified. Privacy was given and relatives comforted. One of us then had to escort the body to the morgue with the porters, carrying the patient's files and ID card before handing them over to the attendant who'd assign them a drawer and issue a chit to confirm that the patient now resided in cubicle number X. It wasn't easy and could be distressing at times. The best thing was to keep busy and follow the senior nurse who knew exactly what she was doing. I knew that one day I'd be the senior guiding junior nurses, so I followed her lead. The thing that struck me most was the silence. You don't speak; you just get on with it. You don't say more than you have to over a body. You are reverent and respectful. Then you put away their personal effects and fold their clothes ready for the relatives.

Seeing death in such an intimate way makes you feel differently about it somehow. The body is so patently a shell and there is nothing of the person left within. In Islamic law, death is only the end of this worldly life and marks the beginning of a new afterlife, when the soul is extracted and interrogated by angels to test its faith. The righteous will go to Paradise, while the ungodly go to Hell. I didn't know much about that, or where my first few dead patients were headed, but I'm glad that I helped care for them in the right way in their final moments on this earth.

CHAPTER SEVEN

London, England, 1959

I graduated from basic nursing training in November 1959, having sat and passed my state exams to become an SRN, or state registered nurse. It felt like such a personal victory and my father – who was on a flying visit to London at the time – was there to congratulate me.

Eventually, though, the work and the winter and the late nights caught up with me and I developed a cough that turned to pneumonia. Dad visited me in hospital before returning home, and a few weeks later – as a special dispensation and because my grades were good – Colonel Crook kindly arranged for me to go back to Somaliland for a month over Christmas. The colonel insisted that the British weather wouldn't be good for my chest and that I would recover my strength more quickly in my home country, where the temperature was thirty degrees. He was right. Eager to spend some time with Dad, who was living in Burao and had recently been awarded the British Empire Medal for 'Services to the Crown', I put on my uniform and went to work in his TB clinic – happy to be fully trained at last. I did a few ward rounds with him and was thrilled that he was finally able to watch me working in a professional capacity, confident that I wasn't all fingers and thumbs. He could see that I knew what had to be done, and he trusted me more with his patients than my mother ever did with her favourite teacups.

On one occasion, I assisted him drain a patient's lungs of fluid, attaching all the right tubes as I watched him nod his approval. I, in turn, was amazed how ably he managed all that he did with so little of the equipment and resources I had grown accustomed to in Britain. With my newly professional eyes, I realized then for the first time that coming home to work in a hospital as short on supplies as his would probably be my biggest challenge.

I returned to London fully recharged. My suitcase was packed with spices and jars of hot chilli paste to add to the English food or swap for fresh farm eggs or homemade jam. My friends in the UK couldn't stomach the paste I ate as if it were Marmite. When they tried it their faces would go red and they'd sputter, 'Oh my God, Edna! How can you eat that?' Whenever we had money a group of us Somalis would seek out an Indian restaurant (rare at the time) and blow it on a blisteringly hot Madras curry to remind us of home. If someone had an Indian friend we'd fish for an invite so we could eat as much as we liked. Not that I wanted to gain weight because whenever I went out dancing I was still keen to accentuate my three best attributes – my eyes, my legs, and especially my narrow waist, which I showed off with a swing skirt I sewed myself.

After a dance, I'd return to our nurse's quarters in the early hours, sleep for an hour or two, and then start straight back at work. Friends who knew what time I'd arrived home were surprised to see me on duty again the following morning. 'How do you do that, Edna?' they'd ask, and I'd shrug and reply, 'I just love it.' And I did. Dancing helped me maintain both physical strength and stamina. I was able to work such long hours without a break because I was young and fit. I also loved my work so much that half the time I thought, 'Oh my God, somebody is paying me for this!' I'd have worked for free.

★★★

My next big challenge was to decide what kind of nursing to specialize in. Inspired by Tiger Monk and my stimulating experiences as a theatre nurse, I had become convinced that surgical nursing was my vocation, but this was the one and only time my father intervened in my career plans.

Previously whenever I made a choice, he'd say, 'Good, Shukri, go for it.' I expected much the same when I asked him about surgical nursing on my next visit to Hargeisa, but his answer surprised me. 'Surgery is important,' he replied carefully. 'But how many patients will you be able to help when you come home? What are you going to do when women who are about to deliver their babies need your help and you're the only trained woman there?' He had a point. I thought a lot about what he said, and decided that I would take the first part of a midwifery programme to see how I liked it. My father didn't push me into it; he just asked the question and let me answer it for myself. Armed with this thought I began to study midwifery at Hammersmith and later at Lewisham Hospital in January 1960.

Like all student midwives, I began with a month-long block of theory classes in which I had lessons on every aspect of childbirth and went through endless demonstrations with mannequins. Then I was taught how to manage admissions. Later I'd be sent to outpatients and on to the lying-in ward where I'd learn how to feed babies and deal with any problems such as helping mothers breastfeed, before graduating to the business end. Long before that happened, though, I found myself faced with an emergency delivery that almost put me off midwifery for ever. It was a Sunday afternoon in winter and I was working in admissions. As usual, I was wearing the white trousers and tunic of my new uniform. The Sister in charge went for her break, cheerily calling, 'Call me if you need anything or if anyone is admitted, Nurse.' All I had to do in her absence was greet any women in labour as they arrived and call Sister. She would then examine them and decide whether to admit them to the ward or send them home if they just had tummy ache.

Not long after I was left in charge, wailing sirens heralded the arrival of an ambulance that screeched to a halt outside. The crew flung open the back door and called for my help. 'Quick, quick, Nurse! This woman is delivering her baby!'

Panicking, I cried, 'No, I can't! I have to call Sister!'

'There's no time for that!' they protested and pushed me into the back of the vehicle. It was extremely cold that day and the mother was a huge woman with the most enormous abdomen I had ever seen. What made her look even bigger were her multiple layers of clothing, including a coat and shoes. Looking down, I saw that the baby was already bulging in her pants. Knowing that it could die unless I did something, I tore off her garters, knickers, stockings and shoes and then I froze. It all looked so horrific and, as I'd hardly ever seen a baby being born, I had no idea what to do. The ambulance man realized that I was unable to help so he stepped in and supervised the delivery as I watched in a daze. Once the baby was born, he cut the cord and thrust the warm sticky creature into my arms, where it wriggled and squirmed and cried. The whole process seemed disgusting to me – the smell of the baby, the meconium, the blood and goo. I held this slimy thing in my bare arms against my starched white uniform and still I couldn't move.

'Don't just stand there, Nurse!' he cried as he got the placenta out and cleaned up the mother. 'Wrap it up. Clean its face. Take it into the warm.'

Sister returned from her break soon after, took one look at me covered in blood and smiled. Almost casually, she said, 'Oh, you delivered a baby.'

I was aghast and replied, 'No, I did not! I almost died! I didn't know what to do. The ambulance crew was laughing at me.' There was a split second when I thought to myself, 'What am I doing in this profession? Is this what I will have to deal with every day? Did I choose the right thing?' Everyone else thought my experience amusing, but I was terrified and so shocked by this stinky baby that covered my beautiful uniform with gunk. It was a little boy and, to add insult to injury, it peed all over me. It was truly a baptism of fire.

What won me round in the end was the mother, who was so grateful and apologetic. 'I am so sorry about your uniform, Nurse. Thank you.' I thought back to the old man with the abscess on his face that my father had treated while I held the bowl. *'Don't you ever show such an ugly face to one of my patients again!'* he had told me, angrily, and I knew with shame that – on this my first birth – that is exactly what I had done.

Seeing how shaken and upset I was, the Sister took me through everything that happened and explained to me what I should do next time. 'Grab a towel to wrap the baby up and to protect your uniform,' she told me gently. 'Be prepared, Nurse. Giving birth is a very messy business.' When I finally graduated to a labour ward I was able to watch a few more deliveries and see babies being born in far less dramatic circumstances, but it was still a while before I was permitted to touch a mother or child – which was probably just as well.

Eventually I was allowed to glove up and assist for the first time, and that is a scary moment for any student. The midwife told me, 'Okay now, hold the head. Can you feel the descent? Examine the presentation, listen to baby's heartbeat, and look at the perineum.' There was so much to think about. As the childbirth advanced, she warned me to make sure that nothing ruptured. Then came the crucial moment when she freed the anterior shoulder and then the rest of the baby followed in a rush of fluids and blood and I had to cut the cord and clean the newborn before handing it over to its mother. There was no time to celebrate the new life as the midwife asked, 'Has the placenta separated? Did mother tear? Is everything normal?' The pressure and the responsibility felt enormous. I had to assist with four or five deliveries this way although the senior midwives usually picked easy ones to start with, such as women who had had babies before. Then, one day, they told me, 'Okay, Nurse Ismail, this is your baby now', and I almost died of fright. They were still there but I had to manage it, controlling everything from the pushing and the breathing – all under close supervision. The first time they took a step away I cried out, 'No, no! Please don't go too far!' and they reassured me, 'Don't worry. We're keeping an eye on you. You're doing fine.'

From that day on I had to deliver four or five babies a day to reach my allotted target of sixty deliveries for the six-month Part One of my course, and sixty deliveries for the six-month Part Two, before I could sit for my final exams. In truth, I probably delivered nearer ninety for each period. I had to deliver first babies, breech babies, twins, and attend births with all kinds of problems and complications. As young students, we'd plead with mothers and sisters to be allowed to stay on and deliver this baby or that, even if it was way past the end of our shift. In the pursuit of another case, especially an unusual one, you stay for as long as it takes.

One of the things that struck me most about the female anatomy, which I was by then getting very familiar with, was how different it was from person to person. I never once saw a woman who'd been circumcised throughout my seven years in the UK, so I had no idea yet what this might mean for a delivery.

Another thing that registered strongly with me was how vital it was that the right professionals are there because of all the things that can go wrong. I myself bore the scars of a forceps birth. My baby sister died after just such a delivery, and someone who wasn't medically trained dropped and killed my baby brother. No wonder my poor father had been so angry and upset, knowing all that he knew. Watching the miracle of childbirth over and over again, I came to appreciate more than ever how important it was that I would be returning to Somaliland with my midwifery training where it was most desperately needed.

Just as I had loved the precision of the operating theatre, so I loved the supervisory aspect of midwifery. There was a whole hierarchy of staff nurses, sisters, doctors, housemen and consultants above me, people who looked at my notes and checked my findings. Everybody supported everyone else. That first yucky delivery in the back of an ambulance wasn't the only time I was splashed or peed on or worse and it wouldn't be the last. Membranes frequently burst and I'd get amniotic fluids in my nose, eyes and mouth. Blood vessels ruptured and spattered the entire birthing team. I couldn't be disgusted; I had to take it with a pinch of salt and as much dignity as I could muster – just as my father had taught me. The focus was always on the safety of the mother and the baby.

The medical training in Britain was probably the best in the world and I still consider myself extremely lucky to have had it, even though it was before technology changed everything. We didn't have ultrasound until the 1970s but relied instead on an ear trumpet called a pinard stethoscope, or just an ear pressed to the abdomen to pick up sounds. If there were serious doubts about the baby's head fitting through the pelvic bones then, at the limit, we had the use of an X-ray machine. The sonic foetal monitor that came in later was a miracle. To be able to place that onto a woman's abdomen to allow her to hear her baby's heartbeat was intensely moving.

Throughout my time in the UK, I am proud to say that no mother or baby died in my care, and I must have delivered a couple of hundred in that eighteen-month period, many of them in the mother's own home. Once I was working in the community, my 'beat' was Peckham, Kennington, the Oval and Brixton, and I was usually working with women I already knew and whose pregnancy I'd been charting. It was normal procedure to visit each house to check on its suitability in advance and to arrange things in preparation for delivery day. I had to be certain that a stretcher could be carried in and out of the house in case of an emergency. The home delivery room needed to be close to a water source and have a telephone, and a third person had to be there while I was delivering the baby. Only when all of these requirements were in place could I recommend a woman for a home delivery; and even then a supervisor had to come and recheck everything.

The expectant mother would be sent a maternity pack with rubber sheets, absorbent pads, and brown paper for wrapping the debris in, or we'd use old newspapers. They were also given a cash grant for essentials such as nappies or a cot, and a cardboard box of other basic supplies for the day of the delivery, which they weren't allowed to open until one of us said so. Because babies don't always come on the day they are expected, I sometimes had to deal with a birth when the attending midwife wasn't on

duty or perhaps delivering another mother somewhere else. As
the substitute, this meant I'd be delivering somebody that I had
never met in a place I had never been to before, and first I had
to get there.

When I signed in for my midwifery class they asked me if I had
a car and a driving licence. The answer was no.

'Do you have a bicycle?' they asked.

'No.'

'Are you prepared to walk?'

'Yes.' If I'd said no then I wouldn't have been accepted. Once
on duty, I'd be given the address of the mother, her case file and
a road map. I'd collect my bag, and head to the local train station
or bus stop. On the first few occasions I used public transport and
walked, but soon realized that this wasn't getting me there quickly
enough. Plus the addresses were rarely adjacent to good transport
links. Once or twice I hailed a cab, but that was too expensive
and I never had enough money. In the end I found out that the
nurse's home rented bicycles for £1 a month, but everyone else
had already chosen theirs and there was only one left. When I saw
it, I understood why. I called it 'Rusty' and it made so much noise
that you could hear me coming two streets away.

When the chain broke (and it often did), I had to fix it. If there
was a puncture, I had to sort it myself. Rusty was my responsibility
and I had to take good care of it because if it was lost, stolen or
damaged then I would have to pay. With two baskets front and
back, I put the baby resuscitation bag in the front, the delivery
kit in the rear and carried a backpack as well.

It was scary cycling through London not knowing where to
go, especially at night in the rain and the snow. I had my little
yellow A–Z and would stop under a lamppost or study it with
my torch to get my bearings. Sometimes, I'd be looking for a

tenement building and other times a council house. I never once delivered a baby in a mansion. Even when I found the street, it wasn't always easy to find the right number and, in the middle of the night, I'd peer through the darkness or the London fog to look for the only window with lights blazing.

I never once suffered any aggression or threats. On the contrary, there seemed to be an unwritten rule of respect regarding midwives in those days. Very often people came up to me and asked, 'Nurse, are you lost? What are you looking for?' They were always helpful, especially the policemen with whom we had a good rapport. In my head, the clock was ticking. There was a woman in labour who needed me, so every second counted. I might get there too late. The baby might choke and die, or the woman might bleed out or have a seizure. There were so many things running through my mind that I was always in a state of panic when I arrived. However near or far, I was forever trying to get somewhere in a hurry. I never knew when a baby was going to jump out without me being there.

Once I found the address, there was usually at least one woman waiting to greet me as childbirth usually fell to the women while the men remained on the periphery. I would quickly introduce myself, wash my hands, examine the patient, unpack my kit and get on with the delivery. Every case was different and, for a young midwife, there was always some anxiety. Even though I knew that help from the emergency delivery team known as 'the Flying Squad' was only minutes away, I always felt nervous anticipation as the mother endured her final painful contractions. It was my job to set the pace and to make sure that she didn't push too hard or too soon. The baby needed to be delivered slowly, so that it didn't rupture her, or was strangled by its own umbilical cord. I had to ensure that the child wasn't breeched, and that its shoulders emerged one by one after the head, before it slid out in a messy rush.

Then came that boost of adrenalin when a healthy child was born. It is a combination of relief and joy, shared with the mother. I still get that exhilarating feeling when I help bring a new life into the world, kicking and crying. You cannot help but smile.

The midwife's work is still far from over then, however. Aged just twenty-one, I had to cut the umbilical cord and safely deliver the placenta intact, without risk of haemhorrage or future infection. This involved a wait of some fifteen minutes until the contractions began again, and a careful examination of all that was expelled to make sure that there was nothing left inside. If there was, then I'd have to call for help. Even if there were no complications, I'd remain at the mother's side for an hour or more, cleaning her up, washing the baby, and checking them both over. They were still so vulnerable to catastrophe and the responsibility lay heavy on my shoulders. My care would continue every day for the next ten days, until they were well enough and strong enough to cope on their own. During that period, we'd get to know so much about the family and bond with them, which always made saying goodbye difficult on the last visit. I loved to receive 'Thank You' notes and, of course, boxes of chocolates were always welcome.

There were so many home deliveries, but a few I will never forget. I delivered one woman of her twelfth child, the first boy after eleven girls, and the father was so drunk celebrating that he passed out within a few hours of the birth. In that house, like so many others, my path to the mother was cluttered with toys and shoes, plates, bottles and glasses. The youngest children slept beside her bed so I had to persuade a neighbour to take them in while we got on with delivering her baby.

In those days, we midwives wore a white uniform with a navy blue raincoat, black gloves and black equipment bags. We had black bicycles, black caps, and in my case, a black face to go with them! Having been assigned as a substitute midwife again, I looked up another address, found the house and rang the doorbell. A little blond, blue-eyed boy aged about five opened the door and froze. He looked absolutely petrified. Jumping back, he screamed, 'Mummy, Mummy! It's a black nurse. Are we going to have a black baby?' (In those days, children often thought that babies were brought to the house in a doctor or nurse's bag.)

His mother reassured him with, 'Johnny, come inside. Let the poor nurse in.' I laughed it off, chatted with the woman in labour and prepared for her delivery. As it progressed, little Johnny was hanging around to see what colour his new brother or sister would be. To him it made perfect sense that this black apparition in his home could only bring something black into the world. When his tiny blond, blue-eyed brother was born, as white as Johnny, his eyes almost popped out of his head. As I washed and dressed the baby, I smiled at him and said, 'You're probably wondering how I got you a white baby when my bag is black?'

He tilted his head, suspiciously.

'Do you want to know the secret?' When he nodded, I opened my bag and showed him, 'Look at the lining.'

That solved the mystery for little Johnny. As he ran to his mother, I heard him tell her, 'Do you know how nurse brought us a white baby? It's because the lining of her bag is white!'

★★★

My midwifery course was so intense that there was little time for anything else, so late nights and dances were far fewer. The irony was that there were no longer curfews to drag me home early – just exhaustion. I still danced, of course, and often burned the candles at both ends, but I was young and energetic and somehow managed to survive. For security reasons, we had to give our names to the guard at the hospital gate so that in case of a fire or some other emergency in the nurse's block the administrators knew how many of us were on the premises.

The first time a friend of mine returned to the hospital with me, she gave a different name, which I thought a little strange. When I gave my own, she hissed, 'Oh, no Edna, you must give yourself a pseudonym so they can't keep tabs on you.' The next time I came in, I was 'Nurse Brown', a moniker the guards came to know me by.

Not that I went out every night as before, because I was so busy what with all those deliveries plus three days of clinics each week, and umpteen follow-up visits to carry out umbilical checks, change dressings, remove stitches, and deal with any mother's concerns such as how to use warm salt baths for ruptures and tears. The whole year flew by in what seemed like a couple of months. Everything was so packed and competitive. I loved it. I still do. When my midwifery year was up in 1961, I sat my final exams at St Thomas' Hospital in Lambeth along with my friends. There was a practical exam and an oral, so I did the best I could and went home to wait for two long weeks. If I didn't pass I'd have to do it all over again, and there would only be one more chance. If I failed a second time they wouldn't let me sit for it for at least another year, which would have been disastrous.

After a succession of sleepless nights worrying that I hadn't done enough to pass, I went with my colleagues to the Royal College of Midwives in Marylebone to find out if my name was on the list of those who'd got through. It was such a tense moment as each of us frantically scanned the printed lists to see if we were there. With such excellent trainers like Miss Markham and Sister Monk, it would have been disastrous to fail. To my great relief, my name was there – in among all the other nurses with a surname beginning with 'I', and – next to it for the first time – was my registration number. That felt so good and best of all, my group had all passed together.

I immediately sent a telegram to my parents to tell them the good news, and Dad sent me a message straight back:

'*Congratulations. STOP.*'

That night, we celebrated at a restaurant before throwing a party in the nurses' home. There was dancing and singing, everyone was so happy and friends were congratulating us. Many of the younger nurses wanted to know how we did because they were next in line and would be sitting their own finals in three months.

When it came time for our official graduation from the basic midwifery course, we all had to say a formal farewell to Matron and thank her for our training. Dressed in our best uniform, starched and stitched, we had to parade in one by one to see her for our final evaluation – 'You passed/You failed/You didn't do so well/You have to repeat this part', and so on. We didn't sit while we were waiting because, if we did, we'd crease our aprons. Instead we stood in alphabetical order in a line outside Matron's office (or the 'execution chamber' as we called it), waiting to go in one door and out another, so that we couldn't even see the faces of those coming out. When it was my turn, I announced myself as 'Nurse Ismail' as Matron opened my file, looked it over and sighed.

'Hmm, interesting. Very interesting,' she said. 'Tell me Nurse Ismail, alias Nurse Brown. How did you manage to keep such late hours and get such high marks?'

Looking up, I knew then that I hadn't fooled anybody, least of all the guards at the hospital gate who'd checked me in as Ismail each time I came home late. The good news was that I'd passed with flying colours and was so proud to receive my badge, registration number and diploma, a copy of which I sent to my father the following day.

★★★

Dad and I kept in touch by letter and I was always so excited to receive a new one from him. A particular letter that he sent in early 1960, however, held an unexpected surprise. He wrote to tell me that the family of Mohamed Ibrahim Egal, the dashing young man who'd taken me on a few dates in London and sent me that enormous bouquet of flowers, had now sent his relatives to my father to ask for my hand in marriage. 'What shall I tell them?' Dad wrote.

I was staggered. I hadn't seen Mohamed in over five years and, although I'd heard the explanation as to why he'd rushed home to Somaliland on the death of his father, I also knew that he'd taken a wife – the sister of Abdullahi Said Abby, my fellow BBC reviewer – and had children. When he last came to London in 1958, he'd found my address somehow and wrote to tell me he was in town and would love to meet up. He was staying at the Strand Palace Hotel, he said, and gave me the number. I'd read his note and thrown it straight in the bin, cross that he thought he could just pick up where he'd left off. I had no intention of starting a relationship at that time, and no thoughts of marriage. I was older, wiser and stronger, with a mind of my own. I was no longer a naïve Somali girl to be flattered by flowers and pretty words. The last thing I wanted was to become wife number two in an already busy household, and was furious at his nerve. How could he just expect me to run to his arms after all this time? I was also angry with my father who I felt should have immediately declined on my behalf. Usually I replied to Dad's letters immediately, but it took me a few days to get over my shock and compose my thoughts.

'I'm not a camel to be bought at the market and taken home to play with,' I eventually wrote. 'Do you think I am the kind of woman who marries a man that doesn't have the courage to ask me to marry him first? The answer is a big No.' That was the end of that.

At this Dad understood how much Mohamed's proposal had angered me, and declined the offer on my behalf. We both agreed that, at the very least, my would-be suitor should have come to me first. Sensing my hostility, my father never raised the subject with me again.

By this time, Mohamed had given up running his father's business and was now a nationalist politician, which was his true passion. In 1958, he took his seat on the country's legislative council, and in 1959 became the Leader of Government Business, with a view to becoming the Prime Minister to whom the British would be handing over Somaliland the following year. Ours was one of many African countries breaking away from colonial rule and the separation from the UK had been years in the negotiating. The designated date of 26 June 1960 would soon arrive, with a six-month transition period immediately afterwards; and Mohamed would be one of the key players. None of that impressed me, though. I was far too busy working and studying to entertain the idea of becoming anyone's wife, least of all that of a career politician. Besides, I was having far too much fun with my Somali friends who – like me – were all graduating from their studies. There were probably about a hundred Somalis studying or training in the UK during my time there, quite apart from the older communities of sailors and labourers who'd settled there after two world wars. Among the Somalilanders I knew in London were several who would go on to play leading roles in government and politics. Many of us studying in the UK became political leaders, for instance, Mohamed Ibrahim Egal and Ahmed Mohamed Mohamoud Silaanyo became presidents of Somaliland, others became ambassadors, government ministers. Two of us became foreign ministers, others senior heads of government departments, while several joined the United Nations. This was a tangible way Britain prepared the elite of the country for our Independence. This was far removed from the way in which Italy prepared the elite of former Italian Somalia. It was a very exciting time for our country because independence from the British loomed for the first time in more than seventy years of rule and everyone knew it would create great opportunities to make a name for themselves.

The spirit among these young men was highly competitive. We were all in the UK for a relatively short time and our selection had been rigorous. The British weren't willing to support anyone on a scholarship who was likely to waste their money, so we all had to focus and keep a clear career path in mind. Despite our individual ambitions, however, we formed a close-knit community. We were there for each other. We were like a family – they were my brothers and we always celebrated special occasions together. Whenever there were any official graduation ceremonies I was invited. None of us had much family in the UK so as a distant cousin or at least fellow student I'd be asked instead and was more than happy to help mark these important rites of passage.

'Please, Edna, could you wear your traditional nomad's dress?' they'd ask, proud to have fellow Somalis to show off to their English friends. I was happy to do so, and they appreciated the effort. Adorned in my long white dress, I went to places as far afield as Cheltenham College, Durham University, and to Sandhurst military academy where I was delighted to attend the graduation of one of my childhood playmates Hassan Kayd, who'd trained as an Army officer and was itching to get home and take a commission in the Somali Army. That was such a wonderful day, so full of British pomp and ceremony. There was a military band playing rousing music and a formal luncheon with speeches, and everyone was very happy. Hassan looked very handsome in his khaki uniform as he marched with the other cadets and received his pips from some minor member of the royal family.

I was also frequently invited to receptions at East Africa House near Marble Arch, as well as at a grand Knightsbridge residence: Number 1 Hans Crescent, an address behind the famous Harrods department store – another place that was used for overseas students. Gaining confidence, I found myself able to converse with almost anyone I met.

To my delight, my father came to visit me three times during my seven years in London, staying for several weeks. My mother never once accompanied him. These visits gave me rare time alone with him away from his constant duties. I knew that he came to see me primarily but also to buy supplies for his hospital, meet with his British superiors (no doubt to appeal for more funding and equipment) and – as I later discovered – for medical check-ups. He looked well, if a little tired, but I put that down to his workload and the tortuous journey. We spent a lot of time talking about my training and he would ask me many questions. I never doubted that he was pleased with my progress and that meant everything.

Better still, he bought me things I needed, so if I made a list of the textbooks I required he'd take me to a bookshop and buy me them. He would also look me over and inform me that my coat wasn't warm enough or that I should have more sweaters, better shoes or a warmer scarf. Then he'd take me to a store and buy me whatever he felt I required. Whenever Dad was in London he enjoyed reconnecting with some of the Somali boys whose families he knew well, or who he'd met through their shared love of sports. He was keen to know the kind of people I was associating with. I guess it was his way of spying on me, but I was happy to introduce them to him and show them that I also had a family. I took him to several functions and introduced him to my Somali and English friends and their families. Father especially wanted to thank all those who'd kindly invited me to their weddings or to their homes for weekends and holidays. So that he could return the hospitality they'd extended to his daughter, before he flew back home, he hired a large private room in his favourite London hotel, the Cumberland near Marble Arch, and arranged a table for up to thirty people at which he hosted a great dinner for everyone I cared to invite. They were wonderful evenings and he made me feel like a princess.

★★★

After finishing my course in midwifery, I decided I needed to learn something about hospital management, which had never been part of my training. Even though I'd been around hospitals for much of my life I'd never been shown how to run one, which would be vital for when I built my own.

I thought to myself, 'I still cannot run anything. I've never supervised anybody, or planned and directed a health facility on my own. I don't even know anything about managing a hospital ward. I only know what to do when somebody else tells me to.' Once I went home, I knew that I'd likely be placed in charge of entire departments and that people would be expecting big things of me.

When the British would finally leave Somaliland on 1 January 1961, there would only be a handful of qualified Somalis left within the health sector. After that we'd be on our own. Excited as I was by the prospect of freedom from colonial rule, I knew that I needed to extend my training. This was an unusual request because my scholarship had officially ended once I'd qualified and achieved all that I'd been sent to do. All the other nurses went off to be nurses, but I had to convince the Colonial Office that I needed to remain in England for six more months.

Colonel Crook, my ally and my friend, understood my request and endorsed it. He knew that I wanted to learn how to lead people and needed to acquire these additional supervisory skills. Proud as he was of me, though, my father was very impatient to have me back. He was wise enough to know that losing British support would have a dramatic effect on his hospital, staff and resources. In his increasingly tense letters to me, he'd write, 'When are you coming home? You are desperately needed here.'

With Colonel Crook's support, I stayed on to learn how to manage staff and become a buffer between sisters and the junior nurses. I did the rounds with the doctors and helped decide on diets and which ward to place which patient. I had to keep a close eye on supplies and check what we needed to order in. It was my job to ensure that the equipment wasn't faulty, was of good quality and wasn't stolen. I had to deal with staffing crises and be firm with the less experienced nurses to ensure they were providing the correct care for the patients, who always came first. Essentially, I was trained to be a bully.

In London, we Somalilanders celebrated our independence with a big party at East Africa House. We were young and foolish and we didn't know any better. My personal experience of the British had been nothing but positive, as my father and I had been trained and nurtured by them, but we were a patriotic nation and wanted to taste independence for ourselves. In another twist of fate, it was Mohamed Egal who signed the documents that freed us from the British. British Somaliland, first established in the 1880s, became the independent and sovereign State of Somaliland on 26 June 1960, and – less than a week later – part of the Somali Republic when we united with our neighbour the former Italian Somalia, which had been granted its independence soon after ours. Five days later, Mohamed became the new republic's first Prime Minister, on the frontline of politics – which was exactly where he wanted to be.

We young Somalis were euphoric, as this felt like the dawning of a new era in the troubled history of our country. The Act of Union, which was never ratified by the parliaments of the two sovereign Somali countries, led to the creation of the new Somali Republic in what was hoped would be a five-nation union of all Somali-speaking regions including French Somaliland, the Northeastern Province of Kenya, and the Ogaden buffer zone known as the Reserved Area in eastern Ethiopia. A new flag was devised – blue with a white five-pointed star to represent the five members – although none of the others ever joined us once they saw how badly the unification between British Somaliland and Italian Somalia went. Little did we know then that our connection with Somalia – and the world's inability to differentiate between us – would for ever haunt us and give us deep cause for regret.

With all this going on at home and having finished my hospital administration course, my next dream, of training to be an operating theatre nurse under Tiger Monk or someone like her, did not sit well with my father. I knew how helpful this training would be in the new republic, but I also sensed that it wouldn't be popular with Dad, as it would extend my stay in the UK by another year. As I predicted, he was adamant that I return home immediately, so somewhat reluctantly I agreed. With money in my pocket I finally caught the slow boat, having been away since October 1954 – a total of seven years. I had a lot of time on that ship to reflect on my years in London and the life that lay ahead of me. At twenty-three years old, I still imagined myself working side-by-side with my father and helping him create the kind of healthcare that our newly independent country deserved. In the back of my mind, I'd never lost my childhood dream that I would one day build him a hospital. In spite of my youth, a template was being slowly created in my head of just what I'd expect from the medical establishment of my dreams.

Apart from my nursing training, I think what I gained most from my British training was confidence. It didn't come all at once, and I certainly had my trials and disappointments, but what I realize now is how important it was to have others believe in me when I was having self-doubts. My father had never stopped believing in me, and plenty of people since had gone out of their way to support and encourage me. They included everyone from Dr Ashe to Miss Udell, Miss Markham to Colonel Crook to Tiger Monk, not to mention the dozens of others who'd patiently imparted their invaluable knowledge and left me with skills that I still use to this day.

Having been taught by the best, I felt invincible as I placed my feet back on Somali soil, ready to get on with the job. I was incredibly excited about a future that seemed to be shiny and new.

CHAPTER EIGHT

Hargeisa, The Somali Republic, 1960

My father was waiting to greet me at Hargeisa airport when I flew the last leg home from Aden on 9 August 1961. 'Welcome to our new country, Shukri,' he told me, beaming, and I almost cried with happiness upon hearing the name only he ever called me.

Dad had taken some time off from the hospital where he was working in Burao and he and Mum had arranged a big feast to celebrate my return. It was lovely to see everyone again, including Farah and my baby sister Asha, who were both home from school that summer and whom I hadn't seen in a couple of years. Kindly, Dad had invited most of our relatives, which meant a lot of mouths to feed. Like him, I wanted them to see for themselves that the wayward Adan Ismail daughter had returned in one piece and I enjoyed impressing the naysayers who swore I'd never return. There I was, in flesh and blood, not only back but ready to start work in the country that had a new name and a new future. Standing alongside to my father at that feast – a man who was twelve inches taller than me – I felt eight feet tall.

After the celebrations were over, I rose early the next morning and went with Dad to the office of Mohamed Aidid, the Director of Medical Services for the region, and a former student of his. I shook Mr Aidid's hand, sat down in his office, and listened as he explained from behind his huge desk that our National Ministry of Health was now based in Mogadishu, the former capital of Italian Somalia, which was now our capital too.

When it was my turn to speak I told him, 'I am very happy to be reporting for duty, sir. What would you like me to do first?'

'Go to work,' he replied with a shrug.

That was my first shock. I expected him to explain my list of responsibilities and salary, as they would have done in England.

Seeing my hesitation, he added, 'Just do what you're trained to do – go to the hospital and nurse the sick.' There was a pause before he asked, 'You *are* trained, aren't you?'

'Yes, of course,' I faltered, 'but where would you like me to start?'

'At the hospital, where else?'

I was flabbergasted. In the UK I'd have been given a job description, assigned to a specific department, and connected to a staff member who'd provide me with some orientation – the kinds of directives I'd been receiving for seven years.

'But what is my position?'

'We'll have to wait and see. The Ministry will tell us in due course.'

'And who is supervising me?'

He shrugged again.

'What will be my working hours? What's my salary? What about my uniform?'

Frowning, he looked from my father to me as if to say, 'Why is she asking all these questions?'

Impatient, he replied, 'I don't know', and stood to indicate that our time was up. 'You don't need to wear a uniform if you don't want to.'

My jaw dropped. This was unlike anything I'd experienced

and seemed highly unprofessional. Leaving his office shaken and upset, I went straight to my new workplace, the Hargeisa Hospital, which was opened in 1953 and had since become the largest referral facility in Somaliland. To begin with, I just walked through the building, trying to familiarize myself with the physical layout of the place. The hospital had beds for three hundred and fifty patients, for which Dr Ali Sheikh Ibrahim, who'd trained in Scotland as the first Somali MD, was the sole physician in charge of everything from the outpatients unit to surgery. There were two registered nurses on the male wards and none at all in the female section, only poorly trained auxiliaries who didn't know how to read. By default, I realized that I'd be responsible for every female ward – two surgical, one medical, one maternity, as well as a private ward with single rooms for both sexes. Seeing how much needed to be done, I went home, adapted a white dress as a makeshift uniform, wrapped a little cloth around my head as a kind of cap and went to work.

Dad returned to Burao a few days later and came back every few weeks to see how I was getting on, but he could tell how much I was struggling at first. 'I haven't been paid any salary and there is no direction,' I told him. 'I've been left completely on my own.' For the first time in my life I knew what it must have felt like to be him. In all the years he had worked for the British, his workload had been enormous and the stress levels high. He'd dealt virtually single-handedly with everything from necrotic spider bites to cancer and heart attacks, from gonorrhoea to road traffic accidents and strokes. He could administer anaesthesia and perform minor surgery but was unable to perform major surgery and had limited supplies of morphine-based painkillers and only a few antibiotics. He, of all people, knew what I was going through and he encouraged me enormously and promised to take up my case with the authorities. When the money I brought with me from the UK ran out, Dad provided me with a small income. I'd always dreamed of working in the same hospital as him but everything had changed. Since the British left, he'd been officially 'retired' as a senior civil servant in order to qualify for his terminal payment and pension, but then immediately went back to work in Burao for the new Somali government.

My mother was settled in Hargeisa, and didn't want to move from the lovely new house he had built for us all, so she stayed there and he visited us frequently. Much to her distress, my father then took a second wife in Burao. Under Somali law he and my mother were still married and neither ever considered divorce, but Mum nevertheless saw his second marriage as a shameful betrayal after their twenty-seven years alone together. I wasn't that surprised that Dad had found himself someone new but for my mother it was the last straw in a lifetime of disappointment.

After his TB training in the UK, and years of experience treating lung diseases, Dad was appointed as a specialist in TB, which was a huge problem in our country. Because the nomadic community was so distrustful of medicine and doctors the authorities needed someone from the same people who could explain how TB was transmitted and what precautions they could take to protect themselves and their children. Dad had to encourage people to seek help and not hide their symptoms only to infect others, something that is still relevant today. The nomads often insisted that they only had a cough and needed to rest. They were horrified by the idea of long-term treatment keeping them away from their herds and families, asking, 'What about my camels? My sheep? My wife? My kids? My farm?' Even if they agreed to the horrible injections, the treatment took so long and the steroids

made them feel better and gain weight so that they thought they
were cured when they were not.

Only someone like my father, who was so respected and loved
in our country, could convince them that unless they carried on
taking the drugs they'd have a relapse that would be much harder
to treat the second time around. To my dismay, he embraced the
work and completely devoted himself to TB, which was my least
favourite aspect of nursing. I was passionate about obstetrics and
general surgery and I loved the drama of a regular hospital. TB
treatment was too passive for me and I knew from my experiences
at Clare Hall how dispiriting it could be. I understood that the
work he was doing was of vital medical importance, but I couldn't
help feeling resentful that this new role had robbed me of my
chance to work at his side.

★★★

Back in Hargeisa, as a Sister without official rank or status, I did the
rounds with Dr Ali on the female wards every day and when I was
on call – which was every night – I did the rounds of the entire
hospital. If someone was seriously ill or had recently undergone
surgery, the doctor would alert me and ask me to keep an eye
on them, just as my father had done when I was a child. I was
given a small government apartment in one of two semi-detached
bungalows for nursing staff at the rear of the hospital, but I still
had no salary and no supervision.

Drawing on my midwifery training, I took charge of the
maternity ward, where I did whatever needed to be done: admit,
treat, follow-up and discharge. Working alone, I had to deliver
babies in all conditions, sometime using forceps. I also did all
the suturing. Occasionally I would call Dr Ali on the hospital

telephone for help. 'I have a problem here, doctor. Can you please come and have a look?'

'What is it?' he'd ask, always busy with something else.

'I got the baby out, but the placenta won't detach.'

Dr Ali's typical response was, 'You must have seen manual removals done many times, so just get on and do it!' I quickly realized in these cases that if I didn't act, my patient would die. If I intervened, there was a 50/50 chance she might live. In London I'd been instructed to refer emergency situations to someone with the appropriate medical qualifications. Knowing that the new mother only had me, I had no choice but to just get on with the job to the best of my ability. There was nobody else.

I have never worked harder in my life. Within weeks I started the hospital's first pre-natal clinic and its first women's clinic. I also opened a clinic for sick children, but I received no salary for the first eighteen months. The system knew just how many shillings a female cook or a cleaning woman should get but I was a new species, for whom there was no protocol. The adminis-trators had never encountered a Somali woman with nursing and midwifery certificates before so there was no contract, no appointment verified, and no salary category for a trained female nurse. Under pressure, I suspect, from friends of my father and after what felt like months, the paperwork for my appointment was finally drawn up and sent to Mogadishu for approval by the new Minister of Health. Still nothing happened. And I wasn't the only one. Several other professionals I knew were experiencing the same kinds of frustrations and lengthy delays. The feeling was that those in Mogadishu hoped that we'd give up and go back to England, abandoning our part of the country so that they could do what they wanted with it.

The new government we had such high hopes for, which had

been eager to capitalize on our thriving import/export trade in camels, frankincense and myrrh, had been against those of us from Somaliland from the start. Politicians from the former Italian Somalia had tricked Mohamed Egal and his cabinet members into leaving town so that they could push the unification vote through parliament in their absence – amended to their advantage of course – and the unification contract was never formally ratified. Strictly speaking, our union was illegal and yet the government blatantly continued to favour those men from its preferred clans in Italian Somalia. I was triply cursed, being from the Isaaq clan, a woman and from Somaliland.

My case eventually went before the new parliament, where they discussed what should be done about the first woman recommended for a senior civil service position. I can just imagine the debate: 'Why are you pushing us to give a higher salary to this woman than we give to the cleaners or the auxiliaries at the hospital? What is this woman going to do for mothers who are delivering? Even our camels give birth without someone fanning them with their midwifery diploma.' My suggested salary scale was 'C53' which carried a wage of 1,050 shillings per month (the equivalent of $166). Because they knew I was paying no rent and eating meals with my family, their argument was, 'What is she going to do with a salary of 1,050 shillings a month? It is too much to pay a woman!' Or they'd complain, 'Why is Adan Doctor allowing his daughter to work in a hospital? Isn't he ashamed? He doesn't need the money. And who will ever marry this woman? He is killing her and destroying her reputation.' Once again, nothing was decided.

It is hard today to imagine the hostility towards me working, but back then people would think it perfectly acceptable to come up to me and say, 'Look, Edna, what you are doing is not normal, it will bring a bad name to your family.' Others would tell me, 'Your father is too tolerant. Make it easier for him and just stay at home and avoid putting him in such an awkward position.' Similarly, they told my mother, 'Your husband is crazy allowing your daughter to work in a hospital. You should have more sense than that. If your daughter brings disgrace to the family, you will be blamed for it.'

As well as fending for myself and coping with the long hours in a hospital where I had little support, I felt so much pressure, from the outside telling me not to work, and from the inside where three hundred or so patients needed my care. Having lived away from Somaliland almost continually since I was eight years old (and especially after London) I was finding it hard to readjust to the lack of organization, which was worse than ever since independence. My beloved country was in chaos and I was just another of its marginalized citizens. People in Hargeisa were already speaking nostalgically about happier days under British rule. There were songs written about that and a growing movement against unification, with a view to reinstating our independence from Somalia.

I wasn't involved in any of that. I hardly had time to breathe most days. My biggest battle was adjusting to the state of the healthcare system in our new country. The hospital supplies were running out and we had no means or even a system in place to replenish them. It was worse than when I'd helped my father as a child. There may not have been an abundance of necessary items in the 1940s and 50s, but we did have the basics and there was at least a functioning ordering system. By 1961, the differences were stark. Instead of throwing away old and torn rubber gloves we had to save them and cut out pieces to patch the better ones with glue. There were no new syringes or fluid bags so we had to re-use them, boiling everything to try to keep them sterilized.

Tiger Monk would have been horrified. Not once did I consider fleeing back to London, though. The challenge of dealing with these shortages, along with the ongoing misogyny and the multiple problems of our fledgling republic, only made me want to stay and help fix things. Besides, I knew that if I stopped working or pushing for my appointment, then the door would remain closed to other Somali women for ever. I was lucky. I could wait for my salary because I had the financial means – my father was willing to support me for as long as he had to. The woman who came after me probably wouldn't have that kind of insurance behind her. I had to hold on to my position for her, for the future. I refused to give up.

★★★

My other big problem was establishing my credibility with the people of Hargeisa. I may have been *Ina Adan Dhakhtar* – Adan Doctor's daughter – but I was also a wilful young woman who'd defied convention. Those who thought I'd never return from London were now convinced I wouldn't stay. One event above all others helped cement my reputation.

I had only been home a few months and was still multi-tasking when my father's cousin woke me at dawn one morning. 'Come quickly,' he said. 'Khayria needs you!'

'Who? Where is she?'

'In her house.'

'No,' I protested. 'She has to come to the hospital!'

He shook his head. 'You don't understand, Edna. This is Khayria. She is a powerful woman. You must go to her. Besides, she cannot be moved.'

I dressed quickly and rushed out of the door with him, stopping

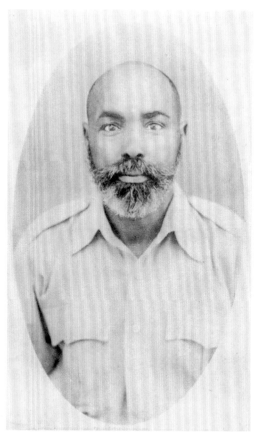

My grandfather
Yusuf Dualeh
Amareh. He
fought in both
world wars and
later became
Postmaster
of British
Somaliland.

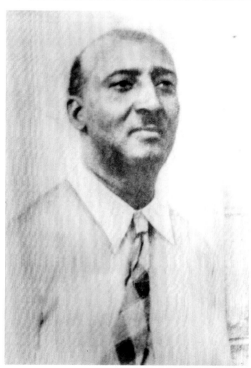

My father Adan
Ismail Guleed,
BEM. He was
the most senior
Somali Medical
Assistant in British
Somaliland.

My third year as
a student nurse at
the West London
Hospital.

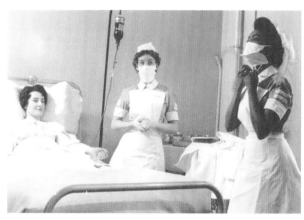

Aged seventeen, in London
where I resided with
Mr Rogers and his family.

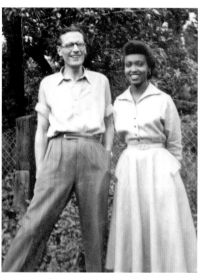

In military fatigues during
'boot camp' in Somalia, 1976.

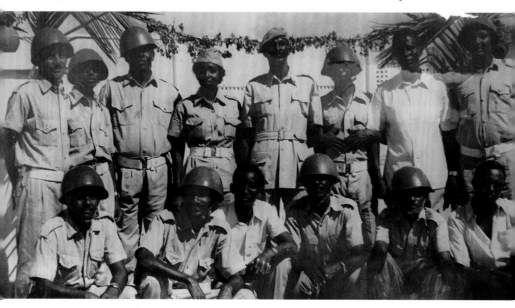

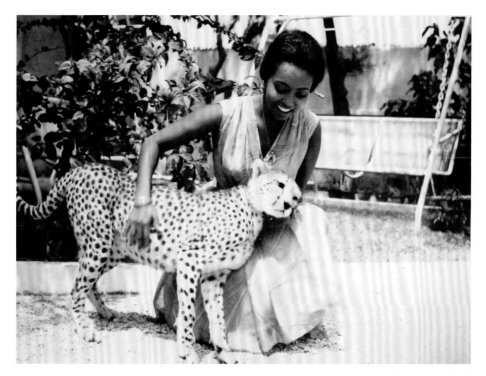

Sanu, my 'Cheetah baby' killed by soldiers after the 1969 Marxist Revolution.

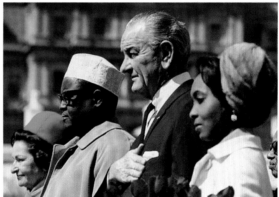

Welcomed by President Lyndon B. Johnson and First Lady Claudia Alta to the White House during the State Visit, 1968.

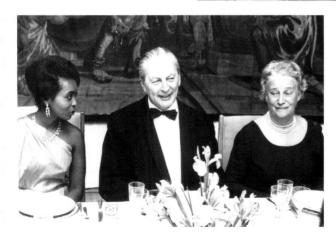

Chancellor Kurt Georg Kiesinger hosting us during the State Visit to West Germany, 1968.

Banquet at the White House for my husband Prime Minister Egal and delegation, 1968.

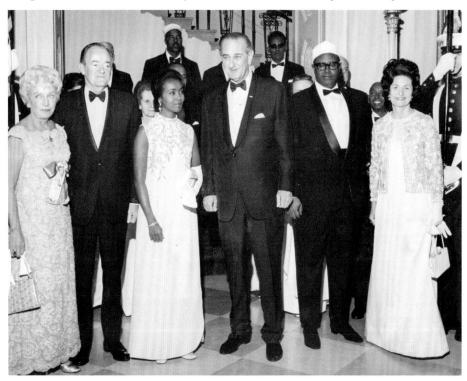

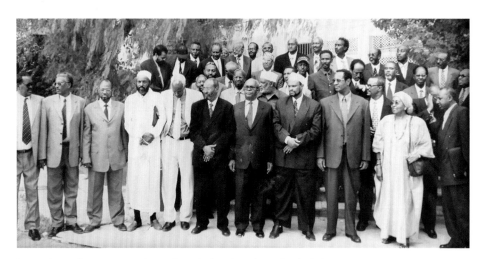

I was the only woman in President Dahir Rayale Kahin's Cabinet, 2002.

Opposite: Her Majesty's Royal Proclamation for the
Independence of British Somaliland Protection.

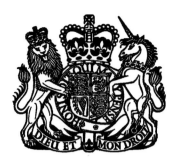

The London Gazette

Published by Authority

Registered as a Newspaper	* *	For Contents see last page

FRIDAY, 24TH JUNE 1960

STATE INTELLIGENCE

BY THE QUEEN

A PROCLAMATION

TERMINATING HER MAJESTY'S PRO-TECTION OVER THE SOMALILAND PROTECTORATE.

ELIZABETH R.

Whereas the territories in Africa known as the Somaliland Protectorate are under Our protection:

And whereas by treaty, grant, usage, sufferance and other lawful means We have power and jurisdiction in the Somaliland Protectorate:

And whereas it is intended that the Somaliland Protectorate shall become an independent country on the twenty-sixth day of June 1960 (hereinafter referred to as " the appointed day "):

Now, therefore, We do hereby, by and with the advice of Our Privy Council, proclaim and declare that, as from the beginning of the appointed day, Our protection over the territories known as the Somaliland Protectorate shall cease, and all treaties and agreements in force immediately before the appointed day between Us or Our Government of the United Kingdom of Great Britain and Northern Ireland and any of the Tribes of the said territories, all Our obligations existing immediately before that day towards the said territories and all functions, powers, rights, authority or jurisdiction exercisable by Us immediately before that day in or in relation to the said territories by treaty, grant, usage, sufferance or otherwise, shall lapse.

Given at Our Court at Buckingham Palace this twenty-third day of June in the year of our Lord one thousand nine hundred and sixty, and in the ninth year of Our Reign.

GOD SAVE THE QUEEN

Lord Chamberlain's Office,
St. James's Palace, London S.W.1.

24th June 1960.

The QUEEN has been graciously pleased to make the following appointments to Her Majesty's Household:

To be Treasurer of the Household:

Edward Birkbeck Wakefield, Esquire, C.I.E., M.P., in the room of the Right Honourable Peter Richard, Baron Newton, resigned.

To be Vice-Chamberlain of the Household:

Richard Charles Brooman-White, Esquire, M.P., in the room of Edward Birkbeck Wakefield, Esquire, C.I.E., M.P.

The appointments to date from the 21st June 1960.

HONOURS AND AWARDS

CENTRAL CHANCERY OF THE ORDERS OF KNIGHTHOOD

St. James's Palace, London S.W.1.

24th June 1960.

ERRATUM

London Gazette Supplement No. 42051 dated 11th June 1960 page 3982;
Before:

Wing Commander William Henry COAST (49035), Royal Air Force, formerly on loan to the Government of Pakistan.

For: *To be an Ordinary Member of the Military Division of the said Most Excellent Order*

Read: *To be an Ordinary Officer of the Military Division of the said Most Excellent Order*

PRIVY COUNCIL OFFICE

24th June 1960.

THE GREENWICH HOSPITAL ACT, 1883

Notice is hereby given that Her Majesty in Council was pleased, on the 23rd day of June 1960, to approve an Order in Council entitled " The Greenwich Hospital (Widows' Pensions and Dependants' Gratuities) Order, 1960."

Copies of the said Order, when published, may be purchased directly from Her Majesty's Stationery Office, at the addresses shown on the last page of this Gazette, or through any bookseller.

At the Court at Buckingham Palace, the 23rd day of June 1960.

PRESENT,

The QUEEN's Most Excellent Majesty in Council

Whereas the Church Commissioners have duly prepared and laid before Her Majesty in Council a Scheme bearing date the 5th day of April 1960, in the words and figures following, that is to say:

" We, the Church Commissioners, acting in pursuance of the Pastoral Reorganisation Measure, 1949, and the Union of Benefices Measures, 1923 to 1952, now humbly lay before Your Majesty in Council the following Scheme which we have prepared with the consent of the Right Reverend Donald, Bishop of Bradford (in witness whereof he has signed this Scheme), for effecting the union of the benefice of

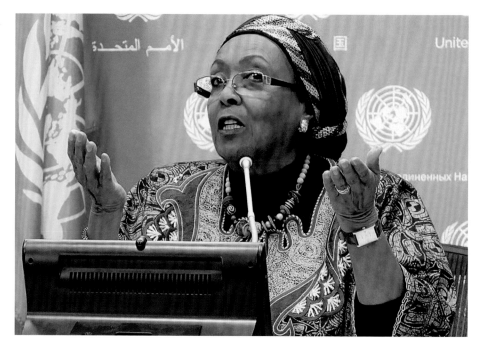

Addressing a session on FGM at the United Nations, 2015.

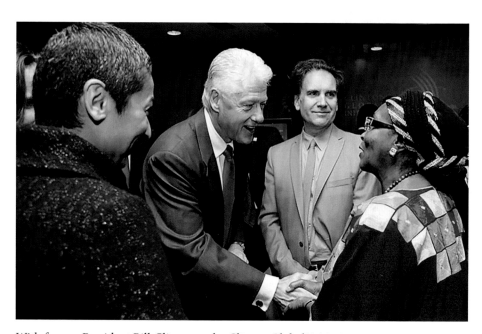

With former President Bill Clinton at the Clinton Global Initiative, 2011.

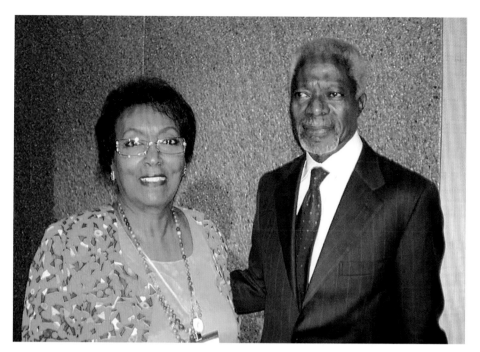

With Kofi Annan, former Secretary General of the United Nations at the Clinton Global Initiative, 2011.

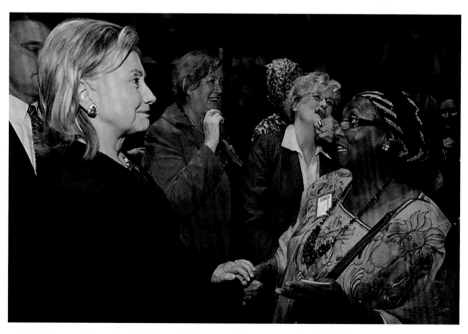

With former First Lady Hillary Clinton at Women in the World Summit, 2010.

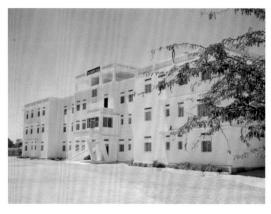

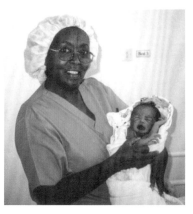

The newly completed Edna Adan Hospital in Hargeisa, Somaliland, 2002.

Harir, the first baby delivered at the Edna Adan Hospital in 2002.

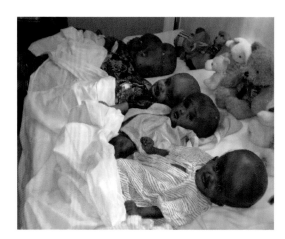

First five children going home after the 'shunt' insertion to treat hydrocephalus at Edna Adan Hospital, 2011.

Graduated midwives across Somaliland receiving delivery kits from Direct Relief.

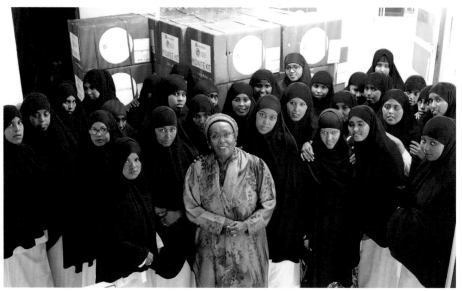

at the hospital to grab my kit, before being taken to her house. Khayria was one of our town's foremost 'spiritual healers' – someone who gives blessings or helps with health problems. People would queue to see her, telling her, 'My son is five years old and still can't walk. Can you help?' or, 'I have been married to my wife for five years and she hasn't given me children. What can you do?' She lived in the shantytown near the bridge, not far from the hospital, and when I arrived some twenty or so women were crowded into her yard, children on their hips, watching and waiting as donkeys and goats stood around chewing whatever they could find. The mud brick house with its corrugated iron roof comprised three rooms side by side and a yard all around. Because she was a woman of prestige she at least had solid walls – her neighbours still lived in thatched huts.

My uncle had explained en route that Khayria – who was in her late thirties – had been delivered of her third or fourth child by a traditional midwife early that morning. The baby was fine, but the placenta refused to come out. The women of the area regarded me with horror when I arrived. There I stood, only five feet two and a half inches, a young Western-looking nurse, weighing 49 kilos, very thin, wearing a short white dress with my neck and legs showing and a white cap on my head. 'She is going to get the placenta out?' one of them exclaimed. 'What does *she* know? She's only a child!'

I shooed as many of them away as I could and told her family that I needed to examine my patient. Day was breaking but it was still dark inside and there was no electricity, just a kerosene lamp. Once I went in, I realized that the sheer numbers of people still standing at the door were blocking what little light there was, so I made them all stand back. In the half-light I assessed the situation and noted the healthy baby lying next to her on the mud floor, wriggling and gurgling, its umbilical cord cut and tied. An abdominal examination found that Khayria's placenta had separated, but that she had a full bladder that was obstructing its expulsion, a common cause of delay and something I was taught on day one in midwifery school. As the traditional birth attendant watched me, mystified, I removed a catheter from my bag, cleaned Khayria up, inserted the tube and drained her of a couple of pints of urine. Immediately afterwards, I supervised the smooth delivery of a complete placenta with all its membranes intact.

As far as the women of Hargeisa were concerned I could forget about the Royal College of Midwives or my shiny SRN registration badge. In their eyes, the morning I saved Khayria when others failed was the day I finally qualified. It was my official start in Somaliland. All I'd done was use a magical little catheter, but I was the woman who did it. That alone was the proof of my worth.

Khayria was, naturally, very grateful to me and she blessed me there and then. 'May God give you blessings, Sister Edna,' she told me, waving her hands expressively. 'May God be with you. May He give you healing hands.' Many people still claim today that it is thanks to the blessings from her that I became a successful midwife. Perhaps it is. Who knows?

After that incident, I was summoned similarly many times in cases that became emergencies because the women chose to give birth at home rather than in a hospital. Another case that stands out was when someone came running into the ward crying, 'Quick, quick, quick! You have to come, Sister Edna. There is a woman giving birth to a creature!'

'Where is she?' I asked.

'In her house.'

'Why don't you bring her to me?'

'We can't. We can't close her legs.'

'Okay let's go.' As my driver took me in the hospital Land Rover to the same part of town where Khayria lived, I imagined with a heavy heart that I would be dealing with a malformed baby. When I spotted the large crowd around the house, I knew it was the place. As with Khayria, there were women, children and cockerels milling around her yard. Word had gone around that someone in that house was giving birth to a monster. Pushing through them, I was horrified to find the poor woman sitting in the doorway of her hut. There was a cloth over her open knees, but she was facing the crowd because it was the only place that had any light.

'These children can't stay here,' I told my driver. 'Get them away.' Then I told all the women to leave us, too. Looking around I asked, 'Who is delivering this baby?' An enormously fat woman stepped forward so I told her, 'Okay, you can stay here with me.' Traditionally a family scatters a bed of sand on the ground and they lay the mother on it so that the blood soaks into that and can be swept away afterwards and not soil the house. Kneeling in front of the woman, I pulled away the cloth and opened her legs further to see a round bulge covered in bloodstained sand. Privately I thought, 'Oh my God! They never trained me for this in London! What am I doing here?'

Showing nothing but a calm exterior, I told my helper, 'Get me some water.' I put on surgical gloves and carefully washed between the mother's legs before wiping the bulge itself. Through my hands I could feel that it was too soft to be a head so I suspected it was some kind of growth or cyst.

The enormous birth attendant, who was kneeling immediately behind me, said impatiently, 'Cut it! Just cut it off! It's obstructing the baby.'

The hairs stood up on the back of my neck. 'No, we will not be doing that,' I said calmly. 'This is *part* of the baby.' Ignoring her cries to sever the growth before it was too late, I put my hand in further and realized that this was a baby boy presenting as a breech birth. Because the mother had been pushing before she was fully dilated, the baby's scrotum had come out first and become strangulated, whereupon it was filling up with blood to the point that it was about to spill its beans.

'Get me a cushion,' I said. 'We have to lift her buttocks.' Once the mother was raised, I waited for her next contraction and told her to push. Slowly but surely the baby descended by its buttocks with the huge scrotum hanging between its legs. Only then was I able to deliver the first foot, followed by the next and finally the rest of the infant. It made a healthy wail and then I delivered the placenta too. Because she had torn badly she needed an episiotomy, for which she needed to go to hospital. 'You must come back with me,' I told the mother, who looked more frightened by that than by the delivery itself. 'There's too much sand everywhere and I need proper lighting and a sterile place to stitch you up, plus I need to give you antibiotics and a tetanus shot and get your baby examined.'

Reluctantly she agreed for the sake of her child, so we wrapped them up and took her back in the Land Rover, where we treated the baby's engorged scrotum with warm saline compresses to bring back the circulation and reduce it. We kept the boy in for three weeks and sent him home with his tiny little beans intact. Thanks to my quick thinking in preventing the birth attendant from cutting off the scrotum, that little boy not only survived but was also prevented from becoming a eunuch. As I told my father afterwards, I had never seen or heard of any case like this before, but I somehow kept my head and made the right decisions, thank goodness.

Dad had warned me that I would be regarded as a threat to

the women who normally delivered babies, as this was their livelihood. Many of them never accepted me but some saw what I did and realized that – despite my youth and stature – I could do something that their years of practice hadn't taught them, and that fascinated them. In time I became accepted, perhaps because I was always careful to thank them for their help and praise them in front of the mother. 'You are a great woman,' I'd say, making sure that everyone could hear me. 'You realized there was a problem with this mother and baby and you called for help. You saved the day!' The large attendant who'd helped me deliver that breech baby with the engorged scrotum became the first traditional midwife I ever gave lessons to. I didn't call it training, though, as that would have been insulting to someone who was older and considered wiser. Instead, I invited her to the hospital so that we could 'learn from each other'. It was my way to get her and others to come. I didn't learn from any of them at all, of course. In fact, they horrified me when they told me all the things they'd been doing.

'How would you deal with a woman who is bleeding out?' I'd ask and they'd tell me how they would wave this burning herb, sing a chant or make a prayer.

'Okay, well let me tell you what I would do.' I'd invite them to the delivery room to watch how I worked. I'd explain why I was doing something a certain way, like listening to the foetal heartbeat with a stethoscope, and keeping everything clean. That is how I gradually won their confidence. We were suddenly colleagues. They went home thinking that they had taught me something, while I'd prayed that I'd got one or two messages into them – mainly keep your hands clean, keep your nails cut. Wash everything possible.

'Is boiled water available at the births you attend?'

'No.'

'Well, do you have hot tea?'

'Yes.'

'So wash your hands with black tea.'

These were ideas I invented on the job. I knew that black tea – especially acacia tea – was an astringent. 'You can clean the perineum with it too,' I told them, warning them not to use the popular sweet tea flavoured with cardamom and cinnamon and made with goat or camel milk. 'And by the way, the sand is not a good idea. Put a clean sheet down instead. You can wash it afterwards or throw it away.' They knew how dirty the sand made the mothers and babies and began to understand. I helped them to learn to find solutions to problems they didn't know they had.

★★★

My father was still working in Burao, but visited us – his first family – at weekends and for holidays. Farah was at school in Sheikh and my little sister Asha was in a local school receiving the kind of education I'd been denied in Somaliland as a child.

Dad seemed very happy on those visits home. He was enjoying his new wife and new life, and although he was working as hard as ever and had his own shortages and problems to contend with, he was clearly delighted that I was back in the country. For reasons I didn't fully understand, he never came to my hospital to follow me around and see me at work, as I so wished he would. I think he felt that he might intimidate me. I did once spot him at the back of a crowded room when I was addressing staff about working practices, but other than that I had to content myself with the few occasions I'd worked alongside him as a qualified nurse in Burao. In hindsight, I think he deliberately stayed away from my place of work to allow me to find the solutions to my problems in my own way.

Every time we reconnected our chief topic of conversation was what to do about my salary. It wasn't just because I needed the money but because I needed recognition and status; an identity and a title for the work I was doing. Dad wondered if it might be worth my while contacting Mohamed Egal who was still in the government, but I dismissed the idea immediately. I hadn't seen Mohamed since our last date in 1955 and had no idea what kind of person he'd become. I knew he had a wife and children in Mogadishu, which had quickly become the centre of our region's commerce, education and diplomatic representation. Mohamed must have felt the same as the rest of us disgruntled British Somalilanders who felt increasingly that we'd become second-class citizens despite our good faith and seniority in the union with our brothers and sisters. Having been our Prime Minister at the time of the unification, he was then demoted to Minister of Defence and finally to Minister of Education. Both appointments were considered a slight to him and to Somaliland, the first of many.

In November 1961, however, he came to Hargeisa on an official visit to the 'Northern Region' as Somaliland was now known, and Dr Ali and I were invited to a formal reception for him hosted by the regional governor at Government House. I was curious to see him but a bit fretful about how our encounter would go. To plan a possible escape route in case things became awkward between us, I arranged that the hospital send me an ambulance at 9 p.m. so I could have an excuse to leave the party for an emergency call.

When I greeted Mohamed in the receiving line, I noted that although he had gained weight it suited him. He was still very attractive and seemed delighted to see me. 'Oh, Edna! How wonderful that you came! I've been trying to get hold of you all these years. Don't go away, I need to talk to you. Let me find you later, so we can have a proper chat.' He did find me a little later on at the reception and began to ask me about my family, but he was very much in demand and was soon whisked away to speak to someone more important. At 9 p.m., as arranged, the ambulance came to take me back to the hospital, where, ironically, I dealt with a genuine emergency.

When I finally walked home two hours later, I found cars parked outside our house and all the lights on, which was very unusual late at night. To my surprise, Mohamed was sitting with Mum on the verandah under the porch lights. By the number of empty teacups and the full ashtray, he'd been there for some time. My mother – who never stayed up late – was fluttering around excitedly.

'Where did you disappear to, Edna?' Mohamed asked with a smile. 'I wanted to talk to you.'

'I had to work,' I replied flatly.

'Oh, okay. Well, I wanted to see you because I'm leaving tomorrow.'

I recall that I was polite but not very friendly and I certainly didn't want to be taken for granted. We discussed my pay situation, still unresolved after four months, and he promised to try to help. 'When are you coming to Mogadishu?' he asked but I told him I didn't have any plans, as I couldn't be spared from the hospital. He eventually left with the promise that we'd meet again soon. A part of me was flattered by his attention, but I was still too busy to contemplate a relationship. My focus was to give back all that I'd been taught in the UK, and help my people so abandoned by the authorities with a health service that was run down and neglected. I had no idea how long it would take me.

It was my father – not me – who decided to visit Mogadishu a few weeks later, out of exasperation and frustration. 'I'm going to fly there myself, make an appointment to see a Ministry official in person, and plead your case.'

Delighted and relieved, convinced that his personal intervention would fix the problem I drove him to the Hargeisa airport for his early morning flight. Putting down his small suitcase, he gave me a farewell hug and then I watched him walk away, waving happily each time he turned. He looked as fit and healthy as ever. Dad was a man who didn't stand still and never took a day sick in his life. I waited to see his plane take off, praying that he'd get some sense out of the Ministry of Health, and then I wandered back to my car. It was only then that I realized he'd left his jacket on my back seat, but it was too late, he had gone. Sighing, I hoped he wouldn't need it in Mogadishu as the weather would be warm.

I went straight back to work and within twenty-four hours Dr Ali and I were summoned to a woman with an obstructed birth in Berbera's government hospital. We grabbed everything we might need and were driven the 150-kilometre journey to Berbera at speed, a police escort clearing our path. We worked with the stricken mother all day and finally delivered the baby safely in the early evening. As was the case whenever we were called by another hospital for an emergency, we stayed a day longer to treat any other patients with serious conditions. There were at least six, so we decided to stay on and do rounds the next day. Early the next morning, we saw a woman needing a mastectomy and another with suspected appendicitis. There was a man with a hernia and two or three other surgical cases. We also reviewed the ongoing treatment of patients on the medical wards. In short, it was just another busy day that took us from case to case with hardly a break in between. The only odd thing was that this was the first time that the surgeon and the nurse were Somalilanders trained in Britain, working just as British surgeons and nursing sisters would previously have done.

When we finished, one of the local police officers told us that a huge American warship had arrived in port and that the doctor and I were invited to a reception aboard the vessel for senior civil servants. We couldn't refuse, so we cleaned up and attended in the clothes we were wearing. We spent a pleasant enough evening before being tendered back to port for the long journey home. As we approached the harbour, I could see crowds of people gathered on the quayside in the dark. As we drew closer, we could hear women weeping and wailing. 'Oh no. I think a child must have fallen into the sea!' I told the doctor, and we both peered into the gloom to see if there was anything we might be able to do. As we disembarked, the crowd pressed around us and, strangely, began wailing even more once they set eyes on me. A teenage boy pushed to the front, ran up to me and asked, 'Are you *Ina Adan Dhakhtar*?'

Puzzled, I answered, 'Yes.'

'Your father has died.'

His face betrayed no emotion or motive and, before I could respond, Dr Ali and the policemen waiting to drive us home pulled me through the crowds and negotiated a path to our car. Turning back to stare at the teenager, I stammered, 'W–what did he say? What does he know about my father?' We were taken to the local police station in silence and I sat in the back of the vehicle, my mind and body rigid. Nobody explained – they just led me into a room in time for me to hear a radio announcement. 'Our condolences to the family of the late Adan Doctor Ismail.' The calendar on the wall told me it was 1 December 1961.

I don't think I fully believed the news until we finally reached Hargeisa at about 3 a.m. and drew up to my house, which was ablaze with lights and crowded with people. That is when I knew it was true. The next few hours are still blurred in my memory but I remember asking my weeping mother, 'How? Was he killed?' She didn't know; they just heard the news on the state radio announcing his death and that he would be given a state funeral in Mogadishu the next day, with President Aden Abdullah Osman heading the procession.

Because of our tradition to bury our dead within twenty-four hours, neither my mother nor I were consulted about where Dad should be laid to rest. We were only women, after all, and women are not even allowed at the graveside of Muslim burials in case they make spectacles of themselves. Only men attend and it is men who decide these things. Distant male relatives we barely knew decided to inter Dad 1,500 kilometres away in a city we didn't know. Aside from the President, many senior government ministers attended the funeral including Mohamed Ibrahim Egal. I didn't care about Mohamed or anyone else, I just wanted to find out how my father had died and visit his grave. He'd only gone to the capital because of me and now he was buried in the unforgiving Somali dirt. How could a healthy fifty-five-year-old man who, five days earlier, had walked nimbly to his plane not be breathing any more? I needed to know.

Three days after his death, I flew to Mogadishu in a Russian military plane arranged by the Army. A driver sent by one of my Dad's relatives collected me and drove me straight to the cemetery, where I was given a number and a map. There was no headstone for my father, and no flowers or adornments. Nothing. It was desolate. In a huge cemetery, a small mound of cement-grey sand marked the spot with a number on a little concrete plaque – 1300. I looked up through my tears and stared blindly at the older graves with weeds growing out of them, and at the twenty or so new graves that had been freshly dug. A hundred metres away, another funeral was in attendance with the male mourners standing around in silence as the body shrouded in white sheets was lowered into the ground.

I don't think I have ever felt as hopeless as I did that day. The place seemed so bleak and monochrome, far from Hargeisa and the colourful life that Adan Ismail had led – as a doctor, father, humanitarian and benefactor. I thought of his great humour and how he exuded life and joy. I found it impossible to imagine that he lay dead beneath my feet. After my relatives finally pulled me away and took me back to the house where they were holding a wake, I was handed my father's suitcase and a small paper parcel containing the rest of his belongings. If only he'd had his jacket, I thought.

Mohamed Egal arrived to express his condolences and said all the right things. He was very kind to me, and gallantly escorted me the following day to meet the Minister of Health and the Prime Minister Abdirashid Ali Shermarke, who promised to look into my pay issue as a matter of urgency. As I returned to my hotel, with assurances from Mohamed that the matter would be sorted, I was grateful at least that in my grief and shock I wasn't completely alone.

It was Engineer Ali Sheikh Mohamed, an old friend of my father's and the first engineer Somaliland ever had, who finally told me what I needed to know. Rather than stay in a hotel, Dad had been invited to stay with him and in the evening the two of them had gone out to dinner together with several old friends from Somaliland. When they returned home, my father told Ali that he wanted to stay up and write me a letter, promising to turn out the light. An hour later, Dad woke his old friend and – with his hand over his heart – asked him to take him to the hospital as he had severe chest pains. My father went back downstairs and collapsed onto the couch. By the time his host dressed and came down, he found Dad unconscious. He and his servants managed to get him into a car and drove him straight to the main De Martino Hospital. It was the early hours and a night nurse came out of the building, felt for my father's pulse, shook his head and announced, 'He's dead. Take him straight to the morgue.'

There was no independent verification of the nurse's hasty diagnosis, no attempt to resuscitate him, and no further measures taken to see if anything could be done to restart his heart. Adan Ismail, who'd devoted his life to medicine and spent forty years giving the best possible care to thousands of men, women and children, was not even afforded the same privilege. Dismissed as a corpse, he was driven to the morgue and assigned a refrigerated drawer. Who knows what might have happened if they'd tried to revive him? How could I live with the fact that I wasn't there to do all I could to keep him alive? I would have loved to have cared for him as he had cared for others all his life. I would have fed him, talked to him, comforted him, washed him, shaved him – things I'd always done for patients but never had the opportunity to do for my own father.

After Dad died, there were several rumours that the Somali authorities might have poisoned him. People said he was too popular and respected in Somaliland and had been murdered because he'd gone to Mogadishu to cause trouble. I can't think about that and I will never be sure but I do know that I found heart medication in his suitcase and that, unbeknownst to me, he had type 2 diabetes that my mother told me he'd been trying to control with diet. He kept this from me, along with a suspected heart arrhythmia that was being monitored each time he came to visit me in London. I am also mindful of the fact that his father,

Grandfather Ismail, died in his sixties, as did my uncle Mohamed, the merchant seaman, so perhaps poor health ran in the male side of our family. It might explain why he let me find my own solutions to my problems and encouraged me not to depend too much on him. Perhaps this could also have been the reason he kept calling me back home.

Dad, you did well by me.

I hope that I have done well by you.

Rest in peace.

Sifting through his belongings and searching through his pockets, I looked in vain for the letter that he'd stayed up to write me; the last letter that never reached its destination. What was he planning to tell me that night? What was so urgent that he wanted to send it then? Why couldn't it wait? I only wish I knew.

Instead of speculating on how and why my father died, all I could focus on was how little I'd seen of him in the previous years, and how much I wished I'd been with him at the end. We'd only had four months in Somaliland since my return and most of it was spent apart. I barely knew his second wife, a woman I called 'Auntie', and I hadn't had a chance to find out much about his new life. I also realized, with a stab of pain, that few people – if any – would ever again call me Shukri.

In spite of all that I had worked hard to achieve, I'd never fulfilled my wish to stand alongside him in uniform every day or have him see me with my sleeves rolled up delivering babies. Perhaps most poignantly of all – I never once had the chance to tell him about my dream to one day build him a hospital that would make him proud.

It is a regret I will live with for the rest of my days.

CHAPTER NINE

Hargeisa, 1961

At 5 a.m. on the morning of 10 December 1961 I was woken by
frantic banging on my door. I had only been home from Mogadishu for a few days and was still reeling from my father's death.
The Hargeisa Hospital where I worked without renumeration
was renamed the Adan Ismail Hospital in his memory, but no
one apart from us yet knew that my father appeared to have had
no money, leaving us broken and broke.

Jumping up and wiping the sleep from my eyes, I opened
the door to find the breathless auxiliary midwife who'd woken
me a few hours earlier to deal with a woman bleeding out after
childbirth. 'Why are you here and not with your patient?' I asked,
still groggy as I pulled on my uniform. 'I've told you never to
leave a patient who's having problems. Call me and I'll come
straight away. You can't waste time in an emergency because
time is precious.'

'The phones aren't working!' she protested. 'There are no cars
moving in town and soldiers everywhere!'

Confused, I finished dressing and hurried to assist with the
patient, who'd started bleeding again. There was no time to think
about telephones or soldiers. The phones often stopped working
and as for the soldiers, I assumed that their presence was related to

the latest border dispute with Ethiopia, which was only seventy kilometres away. As I was tending to the new mother, my father's best friend arrived to inform me that a relative was about to have her baby. 'Then why didn't her family bring her here?' I asked, exasperated.

'A curfew's been imposed and the soldiers are only letting ambulances through.'

That didn't sound good at all. I prayed we weren't about to go into a full-scale war with Ethiopia over the controversial buffer zone that had been created upon our independence from the British. With the curfew in place, I had no choice but to take an ambulance to the woman's home and assess how far into her labour she was. I was also curious to see the situation on the streets for myself. Sure enough, there were no private vehicles on the streets, only military trucks scurrying to and fro. What was going on? Nervously, we drove the patient back to the hospital and I safely delivered her first-born, a son. At around 11 a.m., just as we were cleaning up, we heard sirens wailing and then shooting in the vicinity of the Army headquarters.

Soon afterwards Dr Ali summoned me to help him operate on a soldier who'd been brought in with a gunshot wound to the abdomen. I hurried to the theatre, scrubbed up and took a look at the seriously injured young man. A bullet had entered his side, rupturing his kidney and vital organs. He had lost a great deal of blood. I was just about to remove his clothes for surgery when a military truck pulled up outside and another casualty was brought in on a stretcher. Soldiers dumped him unceremoniously on the floor of the theatre and hurried away. I recognized the injured man immediately as Hassan Kayd, my childhood friend and the young man I'd watched graduate from the Sandhurst military academy in Britain. He was now a two-star lieutenant in the Somaliland

Scouts, a former British Army brigade, and I also knew his wife because I'd attended to her when she was pregnant.

Hassan was in a bad way after being shot through the thigh. He was bleeding profusely and, as Dr Ali attempted to stabilize the first soldier on a table in the next room, I tried to stop Hassan's bleeding by binding his leg with a tourniquet and cutting off his trousers to gain access to the wound. I barely had time to ask him what was going on when another truck pulled up in the yard and more soldiers jumped out. They immediately fired six rapid shots into the wall of the hospital beyond our doors. If they meant to scare us then it worked. A young Indian doctor who'd recently been assigned to us took fright and spent the next few hours hiding in a cupboard in the changing room.

Within seconds, two armed soldiers kicked the theatre doors open and burst in, their automatic rifles aimed directly at Hassan. Instinctively I threw myself over him and heard myself shouting: 'Get out! This is a sterile theatre! You can't come into my theatre with your boots on!' No Somali woman ever spoke to a Somali man like that, least of all a tiny, petrified twenty-four-year-old, but in those few moments I became Tiger Monk.

'He's a traitor! Move out of the way or I'll shoot you too!' one of the soldiers shouted, pointing his gun at me and easing back the trigger. The other soldier stepped forward and jerked the barrel upwards, away from my face, whereupon the first turned the weapon around and hit me across the back of my head with the side of its butt. Shocked and scared, I still refused to leave my patient even when my attacker waved his gun in my face again to indicate that I should step aside.

Hassan was drifting in and out of consciousness but, at that moment, his eyes were open so – still shielding him – I whispered through clenched teeth, 'Act dead!' He did as he was told. Grabbing some of the wadding that I'd pressed against his pulsating leg, I waved it at my assailant, knowing that it would shock anyone not used to seeing so much blood. 'Look at him!' I cried. 'Do you think that anyone who's lost this amount of blood is going to survive? He's a dead man.' Sneering, I added, 'So, is this what you've become? Are Somali soldiers so brave now that they can only kill corpses?'

The two men faltered, so I seized my moment. 'You must wait outside until we have stopped the bleeding and closed the wound. If he survives you can take him to court or do what you like with him, but no one is shooting anyone in my hospital!' Seeing their hesitation, I yelled, 'Out! Get out! Guns are not allowed in this building!'

Thwarted, they retreated reluctantly as Dr Ali and I communicated with our eyes only across the theatre and carried on doing what we were trained to do. There are so many life and death decisions to be made every day in a hospital that those of us who work there are accustomed to keeping calm and focusing on the patient, but my hands were shaking as I tended to Hassan. It was later that I learned he was the disenchanted rebel who'd led more than twenty-six junior officers of the Somaliland Scouts in an abortive military coup. Their plan was to take over Hargeisa and the other major cities until the politicians in Mogadishu agreed to return to the negotiation table and addressed their complaints of discrimination and injustice against Somaliland. Nobody was supposed to get hurt.

Knowing that the soldiers were still outside waiting to kill him, I managed to stem the bleeding and patch him up as best I could. The tourniquet was tied tight under a pressure bandage and I attached a saline drip. The soldiers kept coming back into the theatre with their guns raised and fingers twitching, impatiently telling us to hurry up. Once Dr Ali had stabilized the other soldier and handed him over to an auxiliary, he told me in a whisper, 'They are going to take this man away whatever we say, so we'll have to go too or we'll lose him.' I nodded.

Another military truck appeared outside the hospital and they loaded Hassan in the back. Dr Ali and I climbed in with him, along with a male nurse. All of us were covered in more blood than we had ever seen before or since. When we reached the Birjeex military headquarters two kilometres away, we left Hassan and his nurse under guard and went inside to plead for mercy. The general in charge was a man we both knew quite well, having met him at various civil functions organized by the British before they left. Dr Ali launched straight in and told the general angrily, 'You cannot send your men into my hospital to shoot people! You know full well that this is against all human rights conventions and the military code.'

I added, 'Mosques, temples and hospitals are safe havens from murder.' Together, we continued to berate him, making it clear that Hassan and the other soldier needed urgent surgery and were in no fit state to be interrogated.

The general countered that Hassan was a traitor to his country and his fellow men. He told us that several of his soldiers had been injured and that the culprits would be court martialled and probably executed.

'Let's wait to see if he makes it first,' I commented. 'Then you can court martial him.' The general reluctantly agreed and we were allowed to take Hassan back to the operating theatre for emergency surgery on his thigh. The two original thugs were ordered to guard him but they didn't dare try to enter my theatre again. As I was stripping Hassan of his clothing in preparation for his operation, he reached up and pulled me closer to whisper something in my ear. 'There's a notebook in the top pocket of my jacket,' he said, eyes wide. 'Take it and destroy it. Don't even look at it.'

I pulled away and looked down into his face, knowing that what he was asking me to do was something for which I could be imprisoned or worse. There he lay, a man of principle I'd known since childhood who might yet die for his love of Somaliland. I couldn't possibly refuse. After checking that nobody was looking, I carefully folded his clothes into a pile, found the small notebook and slipped it into the front pocket of my bloodstained uniform. I stayed by his side throughout his surgery and watched as he was wheeled unconscious to a ward. There was no time to rest, change or dispose of the notebook because we were immediately brought a dead soldier who'd been with Hassan Kayd, a young man whose body had been left outside in the heat of the sun for several hours. I knew him straight away as Lieutenant Abdullahi Said Abby, a friend from Hargeisa with whom I had carried out BBC reviews in London, and the brother-in-law of Mohamed Ibrahim Egal. Dr Ali was instructed to carry out a post-mortem on his body, and he asked me to assist.

I had never attended a post-mortem before, and it was terrible to watch a friend being dissected. Dr Ali counted twenty-three bullet wounds, front and back, sustained when soldiers stood over him and pumped bullets into him. The worst thing of all though was the ants. After all those hours left outside without any dignity or respect, the insects had invaded his orifices and were crawling out of his nose and mouth. It was all I could do to remain in the room.

As soon as that was over, I went to see Hassan and begin his post-operative care. His guards wouldn't let him out of their sight and as I entered his room they insisted on searching me.

Shrugging, I raised my arms as they patted me down for any weapons, and took a cursory glance inside my pockets. The incriminating notebook was dismissed as the usual nurse's equipment, along with a thermometer, scissors, pocket watch and gauze. I was, however, suddenly intently conscious of it on my person and couldn't wait to dispose of it. Later that night, when − after twenty-four hours without a break at the hospital − I finally went home for a shower and a couple hours of sleep before returning, I dropped the notebook into the toilet pit without ever opening it.

For the next three days I checked on Hassan constantly. He regained consciousness and was eventually able to sit up, eat, and drink. Everything appeared to be healing normally. We didn't really speak − we couldn't with the guards there − but after an enquiring look in his eyes I told him, 'You are fine, and everything else is fine too', at which he sank back gratefully onto his pillow. Later that night I was called back to the hospital for another patient and decided to check on Hassan again. I was worried to find him restless with a fever so I gave him some aspirin and made a note to change his antibiotics the following day. 'Try to get some sleep,' I told him as I left. It was me who tossed and turned, though, as I fretted over whether he might be developing gangrene, tetanus or some other life-threatening infection. Getting up early I hurried back to check on him and was horrified to find his bed empty. 'Where's my patient!' I asked an auxiliary.

'They came at 4 a.m. and took him.'

I was aghast. 'Took him where? He has a fever!'

'I don't know. It was soon after you left. They wrapped him up, carried him to a military ambulance and took him away.'

I called up Dr Ali immediately and became quite hysterical. I think the shock and trauma of the previous week finally caught up with me. 'They stole Hassan Kayd!' I cried. 'They took him from the ward! He has a fever. He might have gangrene. He could die!'

Dr Ali came to see me and we both went back to the general, but there was nothing we could do. 'All the traitors have been sent to Mogadishu,' the senior officer informed us. 'He'll be looked after in the military hospital. And then he'll be tried along with the rest, and executed by a firing squad.'

I cried then, as I hadn't cried in years. Everything overwhelmed me. By this time, the names of those who'd attempted the coup had been published and I knew at least half of them, many from my time in London and almost all from the towns I knew well including Hargeisa, Burao, Berbera, Erigavo and Borama. The kidnapping of Hassan Kayd from our hospital wasn't the last distressing thing I had to deal with after the failed coup, however. Dr Ali had operated on the first soldier who had been brought in as soon as he could, but a few days later he developed an infection and died.

It was some time before we learned what had happened to Hassan and the others who'd survived. To begin with, they were transferred to a military training camp called Halane near Mogadishu, where they were treated inhumanely. After several months, they were taken to what was known as the 'dead cell' in Mogadishu's main jail, an underground chamber where they remained for eighteen months. Astonishingly, at their two-month trial in 1963 the judge threw out the case on the grounds that these officers had only ever sworn their allegiance to the Queen of England, and could not therefore be accused of treason against the Somali Republic. Instead, they were charged with disrupting the peace and instigating public unrest, and subsequently released. When I saw Hassan Kayd a few months later he asked me directly about the notebook and I assured him that it had been safely dealt with.

He and his fellow officers might not have succeeded in their coup, but their court case inadvertently proved that the Act of Union wasn't legally binding between Somaliland and Italian Somalia and hadn't been ratified. This public humiliation for Mogadishu sparked the first of many punitive measures against Somaliland, which would ultimately lead to the arrest and murder of many of our citizens. The twenty-five or so surviving 'traitors' had their military careers terminated and were assigned to civilian positions. To keep him out of the way Hassan Kayd was subsequently sent to work in Somalia's UN mission in New York, where he served for the next eight years. When he left for America, I doubted that I would ever see him again.

★★★

Wrung out, emotionally and physically, I divided my time between home and hospital as I battled on at work in between helping my mother and my siblings cope with the loss of Dad. As his first wife, my mother had been in charge of the wake at our house, which went on for seven days and involved providing food and drink for anyone who called to pay their respects. Panicking, she told me she had very little money left and didn't know if my father had any more funds.

'What are we going to do Edna?' she asked, on the brink of hysteria. The house he'd built had been rented out for income after his move to Burao, so I visited the tenants to see if they owed us anything, but they swore that they'd paid in advance and nothing was due for another three months. I still didn't have any salary, so we had no choice but to borrow from family and friends and cut back heavily on our spending. For the first time in my adult life we had to sell items of Mum's jewellery to survive, as I had nothing worth selling. She and my sister moved into my nursing quarters with me while my brother remained in the government boarding school in Sheikh, something I was determined to continue for as long as I could. There was no more pocket money for him or Asha, and we had to live strictly according to our means — just as Dad had always taught me. Word soon got out that Adan Doctor Ismail had left his family nothing and from that day on people we didn't even know would arrive with cans of cooking oil, boxes of dates and bags of rice or flour — leaving them at our door. It was then that I realized how much my father had influenced the lives of others, not just me. Every day I saw how much people loved him. Several times a week I heard how he'd dealt kindly with them or been generous with his time and money. He was a warm, charismatic man who seemed to have got along well with almost everyone and never said no to a request for aid, so now they wanted to pay back some of his charity.

Not everyone was as kindhearted, however. Many refused to believe that we had nothing as they'd always assumed that any son of the prosperous merchant Ismail 'White Chest' Guleed would be a wealthy man. What they didn't realize was that war and my father's philanthropy had emptied the family coffers. I'm convinced that he blew his lump sum pension payment from the British on his TB clinic when he couldn't get the funding and supplies he needed, and I'm sure that whatever salary the government paid him was also mostly spent on his patients. Not to mention the orphans and the family friends, the poorer relatives and the elderly aunt who moved in to live with my mother for free. He was paying for everyone, including my allowance and the costs of having a second wife, so there was nothing left.

A week or so after Dad's funeral, I received a letter from a local store demanding three hundred shillings – the equivalent of about £50 – that was owed on his credit note. As the eldest child and new head of the family, it was my responsibility to settle any debts. Receiving that letter was a horrible shock, but I ignored it on the basis that the store owner was a family friend and someone my father had helped financially, and told myself that a clerk must have written it in error. Beside, they wanted three hundred shillings I didn't have. When a second and then a third letter arrived, I couldn't dismiss them, especially when they threatened legal action. This felt like a dreadful betrayal. Furious, I borrowed the money from a relative and confronted the shopkeeper. As I silently peeled the notes into his hand, he berated me for taking so long to settle the bill. Once the debt had been paid, I looked him straight in the eye and said through gritted teeth, 'This is sent to you from the grave of Adan Dhakhtar Ismail', before walking out.

***

Work became my therapy and I threw myself into my many duties with renewed vigour. I was Adan Ismail's daughter and I owed it to my father to behave accordingly. One of my biggest challenges when I first arrived back in Somaliland was to find some administrative staff to help me, especially in the antenatal clinic. Beleaguered there, I was single-handedly responsible for writing down the names of the sixty or so weekly patients, recording their birth dates and medical histories, details of their next of kin, their height, weight and blood pressure. Only then could I begin to examine, treat or counsel them. The paperwork consumed far too much of my time and I needed one or two female, literate staff to handle that side in order for me to be able to concentrate on healthcare. But where could I find such help in Somaliland? And who would agree to work for no money?

It was then I remembered my students from the Girls' School in Burao: the daughters of some of the most prominent families that I'd helped teach to read and write. The very fact that their parents had sent them to school indicated that they were more progressive than most Somalis, so I was more hopeful than I might otherwise have been in asking for something as radical. I also knew that the girls would be bored at home, waiting to get married and learning how to be domesticated. Summoning up the courage, I visited their families – many of whom I knew through my father – and asked the parents if they'd allow their daughters to come and help me. The response was almost always the same. 'Work in the hospital? Impossible! That's not at all suitable for a girl.'

I couldn't persuade any of them to give up their daughters, but using all my powers of diplomacy and cunning, I persisted. 'No, no, your daughter wouldn't be working in the hospital, just with me at reception in the clinic, once a week. The only thing she'll have to do is record the names and medical information of the pregnant women who turn up. That's all.'

The parents would eye me suspiciously. 'You're sure she won't be working with men or touching sick people?'

'No, she'll be keeping records in the women's section. All she will touch are pen and paper.' There was no payment offered because I wasn't even being paid, so I explained that the work would be charitable but the girls would feel usefully occupied. After repeating my assurances to each family in turn, I finally persuaded one of the families to let me have their daughter as an intern on a trial arrangement. When her former classmates heard about it, they pleaded to be considered too, so I returned to their families and pressed the argument. In this way, I finally succeeded in recruiting two girls aged seventeen and eighteen, which felt like a major victory.

I also needed help in the maternity ward – to wash the newborns, check their umbilical cords, put them to the breast, and make sure that they were properly looked after. I had a few female auxiliaries trained by the British who'd been delivering babies before I came back to Somaliland, but they were too busy to help me. If I could only employ a few extra girls to keep an eye on the healthy infants and flag up any unhealthy ones, then I could focus on treatments. I went back to the families and asked, 'Do you mind if your daughter helps me with the newborn babies?'

They shook their heads. 'Oh no! That means she will be in the hospital – a place that is full of disease. My daughter will be infected.' They were right to be concerned. When I was teaching in Burao there was an epidemic of smallpox at the local hospital that killed several people, so we were all lined up and vaccinated. I understood the parents' worries, but I still needed to convince them.

'A healthy newborn has no disease,' I promised. 'Your daughter will be in the maternity ward only, helping to clean and care for babies. I'm sure that you want her to get married one day and are looking forward to grandchildren? All I'll be doing is showing her how to care for her own baby one day. That's all.'

They looked at me sceptically. 'Only the newborns? You are certain?'

'I assure you,' I repeated, 'only them.'

That is how I recruited my first three maternity assistants and, before too long, I was training them in how to do different tasks, alongside retraining the auxiliaries to adopt better practices. Not that this was easy. Many of the older women had been delivering babies for years and thought they knew much more than me – the new kid on the block. I had to be inventive with my instructions so that they'd understand. I summoned up memories of the clever and patient ways in which my father had explained things to staff and patients in the past. I'd had the privilege of working with some of the 'dressers' he'd trained and was so impressed with their efficiency, their knowledge of nursing, and the care they gave to the sick. Now it was my turn to teach the rest.

When I discovered that many of these illiterate auxiliaries didn't understand the concept of bacteria because it was something they couldn't see, I told them that it was a *jiin* or bad spirit – which was something they could understand. 'When you don't trim your fingernails, then *jiins* hide under them waiting to attack mothers and babies,' I warned. 'Good spirits stay put, but bad spirits move with you. If you scratch your head or blow your nose, the *jiins* are waiting, so you must wash your hands repeatedly to get rid of them, okay?' They didn't like someone so young and small telling them what to do, but eventually – and only after they saw me acting in a professional way – did they accept that 'Sister Edna' had some expertise after all and began to do as I asked.

One problem I had was their habit of pulling on the umbilical cord after a birth to speed things along and get the placenta out. This can result in haemorrhage and the unwanted inversion of the uterus from which the mother may die of shock. It took me a long time to convince them that this was wrong and that they needed to be patient and meticulous. If anything went severely awry then I'd call Dr Ali to perform a Caesarian section, but mostly I had to get on and deal with it myself. In general, I left the auxiliaries in charge of the women who were on their second, third and fourth deliveries in which there was usually no need to call me, while I coped with the more complicated cases. As ever we all had to manage with very limited supplies, using cut–up cloths rather than sterilized gauze, and asking women to bring in their own clean linen. Every day we had to improvise.

There were so many harmful customs and traditions I had to battle against in Somaliland, but none as serious as the problems female circumcision created during childbirth. In London I'd been alerted to almost every eventuality as a midwife and taught how to anticipate problems and deal with them. None of my training, however, had prepared me for what I faced on my return. No one ever advised me what to do with an infibulated mother, which – at that time – was rarely seen in Britain. It was only when I returned to Somaliland that I saw for myself how anatomically damaged women were. That was a huge professional shock and I couldn't hide my revulsion and anger. It was also the first time that I realized how my own cutting might affect me as a future mother.

In a woman who hasn't been circumcised the female hormones go to work so that by the time they go into labour their skin stretches like elastic to the full size required for the baby's head. After circumcision, the skin is stiff from scar tissue and adhesions. It doesn't stretch; it cracks and bleeds. The mother is trying to push her baby out through an extremely rigid perineum and a restricted vaginal opening. Because of this she cannot fully dilate, which prevents the natural descent of her baby through the birth canal. This only causes more delays and potential brain damage. Many babies die during childbirth because of this. Their families don't even bring them to us; they just tell us afterwards that the baby didn't survive and that it was 'a bad spirit' or 'God's will'.

Even if the infant survives, the mother can be left damaged for life. If the baby's head descends too far and hits a rigid wall of tissue then the contractions can split the mother all the way to the rectum. In cases like these, they can develop what is known as a fistula where their soft tissues are so severely damaged that their bowel, vagina and rectum end up leaking into each other, causing discomfort, inconvenience and smell. This is a worldwide problem when mothers don't receive the correct care during childbirth. They are exacerbated greatly by being cut. If a baby's head is left too long in the birth canal then the bones of its skull compress delicate blood vessels and tissues, cut off the blood supply and can make the tissues necrotic. This can cause a hole to open between the urethra and the vagina through which urine leaks, or faeces through the hole between the vagina and the rectum. A woman with a post-delivery fistula risks losing her sphincter and being unable to control her bowel movements in the normal way. Living in villages without access to running water they become social pariahs, shunned and ostracised, facing a lifetime of rejection and shame. I know of one young woman who was almost murdered by her husband because he found her so repulsive to be near.

In a normal delivery in a hospital with ultrasound and other high-tech equipment a baby with a large head would be identified long before the birth and would be delivered instead by C-section. Or, if it was delivered vaginally and became stuck then it would be helped out with forceps, vacuum extraction, or other medical interventions that prevent these kinds of tragedies from happening. A nomadic mother giving birth out in the bush who has never been scanned and is unassisted or being delivered by a traditional attendant would have no such help and – if she has been infibulated and cut – then she and her baby are doubly at risk.

I saw these kinds of horrific complications with almost every woman I delivered. Day after day in Somaliland, as I had to cut open my patients' infibulated labia and check their vaginal walls or help get their babies out through scarred openings, my anger mounted. Working alone, I had no choice but to deal with it and try to deliver each baby safely through this resisting outlet, a far cry from all the normal 'soft' births I'd dealt with in London. Every time, the memory of my own horrific experience came flooding back to me. All the pain and hurt and revulsion I had felt as a girl resurfaced. It made me want to scream, but I couldn't. I had to control my emotions. As a trained nurse it is my job to do what is best for the mother and baby without questioning what has happened, but as a midwife I was furious about the unnecessary pain and danger being suffered by the women in my care. That's when I first started to react to female circumcision negatively. I was twenty-four years old and it was a 'light bulb moment' for me.

I realized that circumcision was not a universal practice for very good medical reasons. I wanted to run to every girl I saw and warn her what might happen, but I didn't know how to begin. This was our tradition, and that of many other countries in our region and on our continent. It was all about honour and dignity – the honour of the family depending on what was between their daughter's legs. Few, if any, of the men thought to complain. This was woman's business. How could I, Edna Adan Ismail, a fatherless nurse in a country that seemed to be on the brink of a war, fight something so historic and ingrained in our culture? I suppose what eventually gave me the courage to try was the memory of my father's fury when it was done to me. Maybe if more men had shown revulsion and opposition like he had then more girls might have been spared the experience. I had to find a way to turn my inner anger into action, although it would be many years before I was brave enough to speak out.

CHAPTER TEN

Hargeisa, 1963

On 1 January 1963, the authorities finally signed off on my salary and I became the first Somali woman ever appointed to a senior civil service position. They were clever, though, and only paid me from the date my rate was agreed, not from when I'd started work on 10 August 1961. I had to forgo twenty months' income and content myself with the accolade.

The first purchase I made with my new wages was a fourth-hand Fiat 600 left in Hargeisa by an Italian doctor who'd come to assist us for a while. It was an old jalopy, but I loved it for the freedom it gave me to go wherever I pleased. I am sure that Mohamed Ibrahim Egal had a hand in pushing the Ministry of Health officials into action, for which I was grateful. I saw him again in late 1962 when he threw me a lavish party at his Mogadishu house. He'd divorced his wife by then and was a free man, he told me, as he introduced me to a 'Who's Who' of the city. No one had ever made such a fuss of me or thrown that kind of reception in my honour. He'd hired caterers and set up chairs and tables in the garden, with white-coated waiters serving drinks and canapés. I wore my best dress, which accentuated my waist, and high heels to show off my legs. I also paid special attention to my hair and make-up, to bring out the best in my eyes.

When the party was over, he drove me back to my hotel the long way round, stopping at the beach and walking with me along the Corniche, where we chatted in the warm evening breeze. The next day he wrote me a note, the first of many that I kept for years, telling me how much he was missing me. That night he took me to dinner at a fancy restaurant where it became clear to me that he was building up to another proposal of marriage. By this time we had formed an emotional bond and, although I was secretly pleased at how attentive and romantic he was, I felt that it was too soon for me to make such a momentous decision. I needed to get to know Mohamed better. He was still knee-deep in opposition politics and I wasn't sure that was the kind of life I wanted. I flew home and, three months later, after several letters had passed between us – Mohamed followed me. He invited Khadija, a cousin of his and my mother's, to be my chaperone when he took me to dinner at the members-only Hargeisa Officers' Club, a former British establishment. After our meal, he blurted, 'I am here to ask for your hand in marriage, Edna. Are you going to turn me down again?'

'You never actually asked me before,' I reminded him with a smile. 'You asked my father.'

'Then let me do the right thing,' he offered. 'I am asking you now, and who else do you want me to ask?' At my behest, he sent his uncles to talk to my uncles, who made a formal request. 'Our family is asking your family to grant us this honour.' When my uncles informed me of the proposal I responded, 'Why not?' In truth, I was very much in love. We seemed a perfect match, challenging one another intellectually and sparring with each other verbally. I admired him enormously as a principled politician. He was gallant and respectful and I liked the way he handled things. He appeared to be very much in love with me too; even though

I made it clear to him from the outset that I would never be a traditional Somali wife.

'There is no way I am ever going to give up work,' I warned.

'I know, Edna. You are your father's daughter,' Mohamed replied, his eyes twinkling. He promised that he understood, so the contract was negotiated between both families and sanctioned by the imam. When my husband-to-be paid the 'bride price' we found a house in Hargeisa. As I moved in with my mother and sister in preparation for our marriage, the date for our wedding reception was set in three months' time.

★★★

Mohamed and I were married on 12 April 1963. I had rejected the idea of a traditional Somali wedding in which the men feast separately while the women dance, sing and eat on their own, as the bride receives advice about obedience and duty from her elders. Perhaps unsurprisingly, I chose to have a Western-style reception instead. I only wish my father could have been there to share in my happiness.

Instead of a traditional red-and-yellow-striped *subeia* draped around me, I wore a lavish Dior-style white wedding dress made for me by local dressmaker. The full-length gown, which was adorned with silk flowers, had a veil and a long train sewn to a white floral crown. I chose the pattern from a book and then my mother and I flew to Aden to choose the fabric and buy new clothes for my trousseau. She was so relieved that I was getting married at last that she was delighted to come with me. I had rarely seen her so happy. Not only was I finally becoming a wife but I was also marrying into a respectable family, from the same clan, and my future husband was wealthy and important as the first Prime Minister of an independent Somali nation. It was more than she'd ever dared hope.

The open-air reception was for several hundred guests, including many of our British friends. It was held at the Officers' Club and there was a band and speeches so it was all rather wonderful. The Brits all drank champagne while we Somalis toasted each other in soft drinks, as alcohol for Muslims is banned in our country. My two bridesmaids, Mohamed's cousins Khadija and Kinsie, were dressed in pale blue.

Halfway through the evening, the rain came and pelted the cracked earth in the way it only seems to do in our part of the world. Although rain on a wedding day is considered a good omen that will bless the marriage with wealth and children, it was always a risk holding our wedding at the start of the annual *Gu* (rainy season). We scrambled to find cover as best we could but by 9 p.m. it was still raining just as hard and some of our guests began to leave, so we decided it was time for us to do the same. Unfortunately, the nearby *wadi* or riverbed, which we had to cross to get to our new home, was flooded. Since there was no proper bridge, a police car drove us to the riverbank and radioed for another to meet us on the other side. The only way to cross the torrent was via a rope footbridge, swaying violently back and forth in the storm.

This wasn't how I'd planned my wedding or my departure from the reception, which should have been in the best limousine in Hargeisa. My carefully applied make-up was streaking down my cheeks, my prettily hennaed hands were smudged, my lovely dress was soggy and spattered with mud, and my stiletto heels kept getting stuck between the wooden slats of the footbridge. With the river foaming beneath us, it seemed to take an eternity to reach the other side. Soaked to our underwear, we climbed into the police truck and dripped puddles all the way to our house. What was left of my dress, veil and fancy shoes wasn't worth saving. That event turned out to be an apt prelude to our stormy marriage.

Things only got worse. My wedding night proved to be the most horrible experience of my life since the day I was cut at eight years old. All the romantic notions I'd had about marrying Mohamed – feelings of love, affection and comfort – were swept away in the privacy of our bedroom. The women in my family had warned me that my wedding night would be remembered chiefly for its pain. Having seen for myself the results of circumcision on other women, I half expected it but had foolishly taken their warnings with a pinch of salt.

'You're excited now, Edna, but you wait!' my mother, aunts and cousins told me conspiratorially. 'You'll have to be brave. Don't struggle or fight or scratch your husband. Remember, he's entitled to call on his brothers to hold you down if you do, and you don't want that.' I sincerely hoped that it wouldn't come to that, and felt sure that my kind, considerate husband would never do anything to hurt or embarrass me, but our first night together trying to consummate our marriage was nothing short of traumatic; an embarrassing and humiliating struggle. Mohamed was apologetic and patient with me but, in the end, he admitted defeat and declared that it was impossible because of my circumcision.

Somali tradition dictates that when this happens (as it very often does) the husband has to report to the family that the couple couldn't have sex as his wife was 'all blocked up'. Instead of being upset or disappointed, her family reacts happily to this news, exclaiming triumphantly, 'That's the kind of girl we raised – a clean girl! This is what it was done for. She is how she should be.' The next step is the worst of all. I had to be physically examined by my mother, aunts, my mother-in-law and my husband's closest female relatives. I would rather have had the pain of Mohamed bursting me open himself than the humiliation of this public inspection, which brought so many unwanted memories flooding back. The women – who were all staying in my house for the statutory seven days – ululated as I took off my underwear and sat on a stool before opening my legs.

In preparation for what was coming next, I'd insisted that one of my auxiliary midwives perform the necessary surgery on me, rather than a traditional birth attendant, the likes of whom had cut me all those years before. 'Bring a fresh scalpel, local anaesthesia, swabs, pads, clean needles and syringes,' I'd told the nurse I knew and trusted. Had I demanded that she operate on me in private, far from prying eyes as I would have preferred, my honour and that of my family would have been brought into question and the marriage at risk of being nullified. As everyone crowded in to watch, she examined my butchered flesh before injecting me with anaesthetic as I winced. After a few minutes, and on a nod from me as I gripped the side of the stool with both hands, she leaned in and sliced me open.

In my mind I couldn't help but return to the day of my child-hood cutting, with all the shock and pain and sense of shame and betrayal that overwhelmed me. Fighting back the tears, I waited until she'd finished, closed my legs carefully and limped away from the matriarchs to weep in private. Now that I had been reopened, I was left with another raw wound with all its agonies of urinating and healing. At least this time there were no acacia thorns and my legs weren't bound. Swallowing aspirin, I dosed myself up as best I could because that night Mohamed was obliged to consummate our marriage, which was once again excruciating. As before, he was deeply apologetic. He could see the pain I was in and he tried to comfort me, but nothing can comfort you when you are in that situation. The following morning, the women in the house examined our bloodstained bed sheets and declared my honour intact. It took me over a week to heal physically, even with all my nursing expertise, using Vaseline, gauze and antibiotic cream. The emotional damage never really healed.

Mohamed and I stayed quietly in Hargeisa for a week while I recovered, and then he took me to the Rock Hotel in Aden City for our honeymoon. I'll never forget our romantic walks on the moonlit beach every evening. I have never seen such a moon before or since with its perfect reflection glimmering on the water as a warm sea breeze billowed around us. It was only then, and once I was completely healed, that I felt that our romance truly began.

When the honeymoon was over, Mohamed flew back to Mogadishu as the leader of the opposition and I remained in Hargeisa where my responsibilities at the hospital – and to my father's memory – occupied me night and day.

★★★

Some of my emergency work sent me out of town to the nomadic settlements, just as it used to with my dad. Going there was always an experience and took me straight back to my clan roots. In these remote settlements, the women sleep in traditional huts known as *aqals* made of animal skins or mats thrown over a pyramid of wood, while the men and boys sleep outside. There is one enclosure for the dromedaries and another for the nomads in their turbans to sit around a campfire. The number and quality of a family's camels marks their wealth and prestige, so the animals are generally well looked after. A family without camels is nothing as they are not only symbols of status, but mobile ATM machines you can exchange for money any time you need it. They can also be given in payment, compensation for injury, or as a bride price.

The females are worth the money; the males are mostly for mating and meat. A female camel will allow you to milk her several times a day and there is nothing nicer than camel steak. Camel hide makes the best shoes and is also cut into long thin strips that are used like twine. The nomads wet it and bind wood to create shelters and, when it dries and hardens it is tougher than the wood itself and lasts a lifetime. Camel bones are honed into tools or sold to make into ornaments. They can also be crushed for a high-calcium animal feed. These creatures aren't just peculiar looking animals with beautiful eyelashes; they are a whole way of life. The nomads travel hundreds of kilometres, seeking water and grazing for herds that feed on acacia pods, leaves and grass. A scout goes ahead and comes back to advise where to head next, usually one or two days' march away, and often following the clouds, looking for areas that might have had rain. Townspeople say to never trust a nomad if they claim something is only a short distance away as this could really mean twelve hours' march.

Without any telephones or radios, the nomads have no means of communicating with the outside world if someone falls sick or has a difficult pregnancy, so they try to deal with it themselves, using herbal remedies and traditional midwives. They only call for help as a last resort if that doesn't work. That's when I'd be summoned, often with Dr Ali.

Knowing that every large village has a police officer with a radio, the scouts would hurry to the nearest one and ask them to radio to Hargeisa police station and alert us to the emergency. The police would bring the message to us and then we'd have to assess whether one or both of us needed to attend. If there was a clear picture of the situation then we could usually decide which it should be, but often it was so confusing that I'd beg him, 'Please don't send me there on my own. I have no idea what I'll find.' Then we would go together, taking as much equipment as we could – forceps and delivering kits, surgical equipment, painkillers and anaesthetic. The police station would send us trackers who'd escort us on a journey of several hours in an old station wagon to the village or remote nomadic encampment.

One such night we arrived at a camp to find a woman who'd delivered a baby before we arrived but was very anaemic. She urgently needed a blood transfusion, so we decided to take her to Hargeisa, give her what she needed and monitor her for a few days. I climbed into the back of the vehicle with her and our police escort while Dr Ali sat up front with the police driver. That's when the police told us that the nomads had handed over an Ethiopian soldier who'd gone AWOL from his unit and wanted to defect to Somaliland, a common occurrence. The police were obliged to take him back to the city, so he was loaded into the back with me, the new mother lying on a blanket with her baby, and an armed police officer. Halfway through the journey, the prisoner addressed me softly. 'Excuse me, Nurse. I have a gun. The police forgot to search me and I think they should take it away.'

I was shocked. I could just imagine him showing me his weapon and the policeman thinking he was going to use it and shooting all of us in that enclosed space, for we'd surely be caught in the crossfire. Taking a deep breath, I told him, 'Don't move and don't take it out. Where is it?'

'Down the back of my trousers, under my belt.'

'All right. Don't do anything. Keep your hands where I can see them. We don't want any accidents.' Calling to the front of the vehicle, I told Dr Ali we had a problem to get his attention and then I turned to the armed escort. 'Officer, this man's just informed me that he's carrying a gun and has offered me to take it from him. I'm going to do just that, so stay calm and nothing bad will happen.' Carefully, as the car bumped along the camel track, I reached across my patient and told the Ethiopian, 'Turn your back.' As slowly as I could, I pulled out his shirt tucked inside his belt until my fingers found his loaded revolver. I hate guns; I always think they're going to bite me. Lifting it up as if it were poisonous, I handed it over to the policeman. They stopped the car then, pulled him out and searched him thoroughly, as I sat in the back shaking alongside my bewildered patient. 'Oh my God,' I thought to myself. 'I came here to do midwifery, not handle weapons of war. They didn't prepare me for this at the Hammersmith!'

★★★

Mohamed commuted back to see me in Hargeisa whenever he could, but it wasn't the best way to start our marriage. Despite his pre-nuptial promise that he was okay with me working, he didn't like us being apart and neither did I. Nor did he like the kinds of things I occasionally had to do, such as disarm a fugitive soldier. Eventually he connived to get me a job in Mogadishu by persuading an old family friend to hire me. Joe Galea was a Maltese doctor who'd worked with my father and who would go on to have a significant influence on my career. He had married an Englishwoman named Dorothy and come to work in the Somaliland Protectorate as a district medical officer in 1955. They had four children. While living in Hargeisa, he and his wife experienced a terrible tragedy, losing their two youngest children in a scalding accident. Their deaths touched the whole community. How the couple coped with their loss and inevitable feelings of guilt I couldn't imagine, and they left the country soon after, when Joe accepted a job in Borneo. Thankfully, they returned to Somaliland following independence, to support the upgrading of health delivery in the country, and become an important part of my life. Some years later, Joe was appointed a public health adviser with the World Health Organization, an agency of the United Nations, and was posted to Mogadishu. He ran the Health Personnel Training Institute, which worked with lab technicians and wanted to extend its mission to preparing professional midwives. That's where I came in.

'Won't you consider coming to Mogadishu to help me, Edna?' Joe asked on a visit to Hargeisa that was, I discovered later, orchestrated by my husband. 'You'd be a local educator teaching midwifery to students alongside a WHO midwife. It would be an important job and would allow you to spend some time with your husband too.'

Mohamed was all for it. 'It would be far better if you taught other people what you know, rather than expend all your energy on treating patients,' he insisted. 'Dr Galea has this good position for you, on double your salary, and it will mean we can live together at last.'

The decision to move to the capital wasn't as hard as it might have been a year earlier. The hospital in Hargeisa was in far better shape now than when I'd arrived. Two other doctors had arrived to help out by then, plus three new male nurses who'd recently returned from London, and my friend Jessica had also come back. The outpatient clinic was being run adequately by the auxiliaries and the girls I'd enlisted (some of whom went on to become nurses), and I had trained the midwives in the most important skills. Besides, Hargeisa wasn't the same after Dad died and all my British friends had left. The Mogadishu government gave them

just twenty-four hours to pack up and leave after deciding that
our country's long and fruitful relations with Britain should be
completely severed. Going against all protocol advice, I went to
Hargeisa airport to wave them off when everyone else was too
afraid that to do so would be to commit political suicide. I didn't
care. 'This has nothing to do with going against the wishes of the
government,' I protested. 'These people are my friends and I can't
let them leave the country without bidding farewell in the usual
hospitable way.' My actions probably gave the powers-that-be in
Mogadishu one more reason to think of me as a troublemaker.

When I knew that the hospital was in good hands, I packed
my bags, too and left for the capital, saying goodbye to Hargeisa
for many years. With my brother still at school in Sheikh, I only
had to move my mother and teenage sister with me to help me
adapt to my new role as a politician's wife. It was a wrench to go,
but I knew that I was doing the right thing. I loved Mohamed,
I wanted to start a family, and a new challenge had opened up to
me. It was in my nature to rise to it.

CHAPTER ELEVEN

Mogadishu, 1964

Mogadishu in the 1960s was significantly more cosmopolitan than Hargeisa. Instead of low mud-brick bungalows surrounded by mountains, there were soaring white-painted buildings interspersed with cafés, restaurants and nightclubs. It felt foreign to someone from Somaliland who didn't even speak its chief language of Italian or any of the different Somali dialects spoken there, and was going to take some getting used to.

First, though, I had to adjust to living in Mohamed's house – the grandest I had ever lived in. I also had to cope with the novelty of being a stepmother to four of his five children, who ranged in age from three to eleven. The eldest, at fifteen, was at school in London. When his wife moved out, she left the rest behind in the care of a nanny and staff.

It was difficult for the children to accept me at first, but eventually they did. The first time three-year-old little Ibrahim called me 'Mother' was on a day when we were swimming at the beach and he was stung by a jellyfish. Crying pitifully, he came running back to me calling '*Hooyo! Hooyo!*' (Mother! Mother!). It was a word no one had ever used for me before, but one I hoped they would sometime soon. Ibrahim clung to me for protection. I hugged him until the stinging passed and his poor little heart, which was beating at double speed, finally calmed down. From that moment on, he and I shared a strong bond which lasted until his untimely death a few years ago of a stroke at the age of fifty-five.

I had never had much interest in politics, but in Mogadishu I followed Mohamed's political activities with interest. After he'd resigned as a minister he'd created the opposition Somali National Congress as an alliance between the northern Isaaq clan and a section of the southern Hawiye clan. Their members claimed shared ancestry through a forefather. Somali politicians typically used their clan allegiances to mobilize political followings, and the new alliance opposed the government of Abdirashid Ali Shermarke, a Darod clansman from the northeast.

As leader of the opposition, Mohamed was in constant demand for commentary and criticism of the ruling party and was never timid. He admired and often quoted Churchill, Disraeli and Ernest Bevin on the necessity of bold action, and he had no time for sycophants. He often gave speeches and it was on those occasions that I first witnessed what a marvellous public speaker Mohamed was. People were hypnotized by his oratory, as was I. When they learned that he'd be speaking somewhere, they'd flock to the event even though the police often tried to disperse them or sabotage it.

Mohamed taught me a lot about international politics as well. He frequently met with foreign diplomats and enjoyed strong support from Western governments, particularly the Americans and the British, who had no official presence in the new Somalia any more. With their backing, my career politician of a husband looked set to remain a major influence in our country for many years to come.

While he busied himself with all of that, I started at the training school and also gave practical lessons in nursing and midwifery at a local hospital. It was largely dispiriting work at first, chiefly because my only colleague was a Lebanese midwife who was off sick regularly – or perhaps pretending to be sick – passing most of the workload on to me. Some of my students were great but several were late, lazy and dirty. Teenagers from better-off families, they were spoilt and indifferent with an unpleasant attitude towards me, as a young woman from Somaliland.

They found my classical Somali difficult to understand and most had a poor understanding of English, having been taught Italian in school. Having visited Italy a few times, I knew it was a beautiful language, but I could hardly speak it at all. I had to improve on the little I'd picked up, to not only communicate with the students but also the doctors and nuns in the hospital. If it wasn't for the wonderful Dr Galea, who was a great project leader and extremely supportive, I don't believe I would have lasted the three years of my contract. My problems with Italian weren't confined to work either. When I first moved to Mogadishu, it was one of my biggest challenges in this former Italian colony. People on the street would greet me in Italian, and most local businesses had Italian signs in their doors or windows.

While I was happy to be living with my husband again and we had many nights at home entertaining friends or dancing alone to Ella Fitzgerald songs, we began to have disagreements, mostly about me working and not being home when he expected me to be. 'Don't ask Edna anything to do with the house,' he'd complain bitterly to his staff. 'She's hardly ever here.' Or he might say something sharp about me not being a good political wife. His comments were often derisory and undermining and brought back unwanted memories of my mother's constant complaints to my father about working at the hospital. We were trying for a family and I had every intention of taking time out once I fell pregnant, and of being a good mother to my kids, but I also intended to return to my job as soon as I was able. To add to my list of inadequacies, though, I appeared to be infertile. Mohamed already had children, so the problem couldn't be his. The doctors we saw assured me that all was normal physically, but still nothing happened, so each new month brought fresh disappointment.

The resentment between us built and we began to get on each other's nerves. Some of his comments seem trivial in hindsight, but I clearly did things that agitated him, which we'd inevitably fight about. I distinctly recall one issue that, as I look back, epitomized our different points of view. In the first years of our marriage, Mohamed and I acquired some unusual pets. One of them was an adorable lynx named Pixie, a gift from American diplomat friends who were leaving the country and couldn't take her with them. Later, I received a cheetah from the owner of a safari club in Kenya who became a friend to us both. I first met this man when he followed the hunter and conservationist Don Hunt, another friend, into our home a few years later. 'Meet Bill,' said Don, and I said hello to a man holding a bunch of flowers so enormous that I could hardly see his face. They sat down as I called to my husband that we had guests. It took a few minutes before it dawned on me that 'Bill' was the actor William Holden, whom I'd seen in many films, including *The World of Suzie Wong*, when I was living in London. With his girlfriend, the actress Stefanie Powers, he now ran the Mount Kenya Game Ranch and Safari Club, a wildlife conservation centre and a place that procured young animals for zoos all over the world.

The reason he and Don had come to call was to offer me a sick cheetah cub called Sanu. They were leaving the next day and if they took him back to the bush he would die. 'If he survives, you'll have the most beautiful pet,' Bill told me, staring into my eyes with that irascible smile. How could I resist? I already had an ostrich, a cranky baboon, and another pet lynx named Pixie No.2, who was also often sickly but extremely lovable. (Pixie No.1 had sadly died after being bitten by a snake.) Little Sanu was tiny and scruffy but Pixie immediately took care of him. Bill and Don left me calcium powder to mix with his feed and told me I had to make sure he ate things with fur and hair to help his digestive system. Sanu survived and grew fat, handsome and very big. He was like a pet Labrador and followed me around the house devotedly. I, in turn, loved him like a child.

Mohamed grew to love our animals, too, but was never quite as enthusiastic as I was. He would berate his 'crazy Edna' whenever I bought our animals to bed. Well, I had to. Pixie would only settle if she was sucking on my earlobe. One night she was lying asleep under Mohamed's chair, and when he stood up he accidentally stepped on her paw. We both heard the bone crack. She was clearly in pain so the next morning I put her in a large box and took her to the De Martino Hospital, the same building where my father had been pronounced dead a few years earlier. An X-ray confirmed that several bones in her paw were broken, so one of the technicians suggested I take her to a well-known veterinary doctor in Merka.

Merka was a small port town over a hundred kilometres from Mogadishu. Without hesitating I drove to the petrol station, filled up my Fiat, and with Pixie in a box by my side took the bumpy road to Merka. I was so concerned for my pet, I forgot to tell anyone. The Italian vet examined the X-rays I carried with me, and confirmed the fracture. He gave Pixie a tranquilliser to put her to sleep and wrapped wet plaster around the break. 'You can go home for lunch while this plaster hardens,' he told me. 'Come back and pick her up later. She'll be awake in an hour or so.'

When I told him that I'd driven all the way from Mogadishu, he was very surprised and insisted on making me a cheese sandwich. I sat under a tree in my car and ate my lunch as Pixie slept next to me in her box.

She eventually woke up and after a further examination the vet discharged her. I drove all the way back to Mogadishu, where I found everyone in a great uproar because I hadn't reported to work that morning. I'd omitted to tell my mother or Mohamed where I was going, and the only people who saw me leave were the X-ray technicians at the hospital. My family had contacted all the police stations and local hospitals to see if my car had been spotted or any accidents had been reported, but nobody had seen a thing. Just as when I'd been an adventurous baby, I had vanished.

My husband, stepchildren, mother and sister were all unreasonably upset. 'How could you do such an irresponsible thing?' Mohamed cried. 'Driving alone to another town, through the empty bush, with just an injured lynx for company?'

'What if you had had a puncture?' my mother asked.

'I have punctures all the time,' I countered. 'I'd have changed the wheel.'

'What if something had happened to you?' my sister said.

'But nothing did happen, Asha. I am fine and I am here.'

This argument carried on between Mohamed and me for several days and was cited as another example of how headstrong and contrary he found me as a wife.

★★★

It was another incident, however, that caused a more serious rupture to our relationship. During those early years in Mogadishu, Dorothy Galea became pregnant with her fifth child, which they

hoped would be a girl. Joe came to me one morning and told me
that he'd taken her to the hospital the previous night because she
was bleeding. They feared she might be having a miscarriage.
'Would you mind teaching my afternoon classes so that I can be
with her?' he asked.

'Of course and I'll come and see her after class.' When I finished
work I went straight to the hospital where I found Dorothy in
a bad way. She had been haemorrhaging, was very weak, and
in urgent need of a transfusion. As we were both A-positive,
I immediately donated some of my blood. Dorothy was a friend of
many years and I knew she was at risk of dying. With the limited
nursing support available at the hospital at that time, it seemed the
most natural thing in the world to remain with her through the
night until I was sure she was out of danger, which is what I did.
Mohamed was out of town and when he returned the following
morning, he found that I was not at home and his staff informed
him that I hadn't been there all night. In fact, no one had seen
me since I left for work the previous morning.

Even though I explained where I had been on my return
Mohamed didn't understand my need to stay with my friend. To
him, it was improper for a married woman to spend the night
away from her house. He felt my first responsibility was to our
own family and household. It was this lack of understanding and
support for some of the things I did, and what I perceived as a
lack of respect for my professional responsibilities, which led to
our first separation. Exasperated and after only two years' marriage, I moved out of the house and rented a property for three
months for me, my mother, my sister and our pets. Mohamed
and I remained on speaking terms and he was constantly trying
to persuade me to come back to him but I stubbornly told him
that I needed a breather.

Dorothy Galea did lose her baby, sadly, but she recovered and eventually became pregnant again, giving birth to a healthy child. Joe was very grateful for the support I had given his wife and did all he could to help me after I left Mohamed. Knowing of my domestic situation, he suggested I apply for a job with the WHO. 'You're already doing the work of an international civil servant, but are only being paid as a national,' he reminded me. 'Your colleague is making ten times as much as you are, but doing a fraction of the work. You should be paid the equivalent of her salary, and you will never get that by remaining an employee of your own country.' He urged me to fill out the relevant application form.

I was very flattered, but seriously doubted that the WHO would hire someone with such limited employment experiences and academic qualifications. 'I'm only a midwife,' I countered, and let the moment pass.

A couple of weeks later, he asked, 'Well, Edna? Did you fill out that application form yet?'

'Not yet.' I paused. 'I don't even know where it is.'

He smiled and said, 'Let me get you another one. This isn't going to cost you anything, and what have you got to lose? Just fill it in and I'll send it myself. It will take only a few minutes of your time.'

Mainly to get Joe off my back, I filled out the form and gave it to him to post. A few weeks later, I received a letter from the WHO personnel office asking me for a medical report, a chest X-ray to make sure I didn't have TB, and some professional references. Within a matter of weeks, I was amazed to find myself working for the world's most prestigious health organization. In fact, I was the first Somali to ever hold an international position within the United Nations at that time. Overnight I found myself earning a salary of $2,000 a month plus free medical insurance, generous duty free allowances, and permission to pack, ship and transport one ton of my personal belongings anywhere I was posted in the world.

I could hardly believe my luck. At just twenty-eight years old, I was an officially accredited international civil servant with all the accompanying privileges. I only wished my dear Dad had been alive to see it happen. That was the beginning of a whole new career for me, although – as it would turn out – I was far from done with politics and certainly not ready to give up being a midwife in the Horn of Africa. I had unfinished business in Somaliland and I would never stay away too long.

★★★

Tripoli, Libya, 1965

'Saudi Arabia, Yemen or Libya?' Joe asked me, when the WHO job offers started to come in. There were three positions available and I had to put them in order of preference. I felt like a little girl again, having to choose which of the treats my grandmother Clara was hiding behind her back.

'Not Saudi,' I told him, shaking my head. 'I can't imagine living in a place where women aren't allowed to drive.' As for Yemen, I'd been there several times on holiday and wasn't keen on returning, even as a professional. I knew very little about Libya and had to look it up in an encyclopedia where I read that it had a king named Idris and, like Somalia, an Italian colonial heritage. Without hesitation, I listed my preferences as Libya first, then Yemen and Saudi. I was delighted when they granted me my first choice and told me to prepare to relocate to Tripoli. Mohamed wasn't at all happy about it, but that wasn't my problem.

My first public outing as a WHO employee proved horribly embarrassing. Before beginning my posting in October 1965, I was instructed to fly to Alexandria in Egypt for briefings at regional headquarters. A colleague in Mogadishu graciously offered to introduce me to his family there, and I accepted his offer with thanks. Before I left for the airport, he asked if I would take a present to his family. I made space in my suitcase for the small but surprisingly heavy gift-wrapped box. My flight was from Mogadishu to Cairo via Aden, which was embroiled in something known as 'The Aden Emergency', an insurgency organized by the Front for the Liberation of Occupied South Yemen (FLOSY) against the departing British. There had been bombings and assassinations and when I landed at the airport I knew well, I found it almost unrecognizable as it was surrounded by sandbags, and British troops in fatigues were patrolling with machine guns. All arriving passengers were ushered into a transit area to have our luggage searched. Inevitably, the customs official found the gift-wrapped box. Looking up at me quizzically, he asked, 'What's this?'

'I don't know. Somebody asked me to carry it.' I immediately broke into a sweat. Stupidly, I never even bothered to ask what was in the box.

'They all say that.' He summoned a soldier with a sniffer dog, who didn't know what to make of the package. The bomb squad experts arrived and began to open it. I was perspiring heavily as I watched them peel back the paper, as eager to know what was in it as they were. They finally revealed six jars of caviar. Caviar! This was the second time it had got me into trouble.

After they had opened each and every jar, and scooped out the contents to search for drugs or diamonds or whatever they expected to find, they asked me, 'Do you want to take it with you?'

'No! I never want to see it again!'

After my briefing in Egypt, I went on to Libya and my great new job, earning good money and driving around in a new car, an Opel Kadett. Libya was a young country that had recently discovered oil. There was a British base in Benghazi and the American Wheelus Air Force base in Tripoli. As a UN diplomat I had access to the base, which meant that I could buy all manner of luxury food items, from jam to tinned meats and even caviar if I wanted it, although I never did. My mother and sister joined me after a few months and Asha attended the school at the Air Force base while I looked for a suitable English language school. When I couldn't find one locally, she went to a boarding school in Malta, which had been recommended by Joe Galea.

I spent two and a half very happy years in Libya. I started the training of midwives and introduced a new curriculum. There was an excellent WHO representative there, Dr Rafik Khan, a retired colonel from Pakistan, and two other WHO midwives from Syria, neither of whom spoke English well. Seeing that I was fluent they'd tell me, 'Edna, your English is better. You write', leaving me to draw up all the reports. When Dr Rafik found out, he said, 'If you are doing that job too, you should get the grade.' I went from being a Nurse–Midwife Educator to Nursing Services Administrator. Life was good. I found a nice house in an orchard of mandarin and orange trees on what had once been an Italian–owned farm. I made bookshelves and painted the flat in the colours I liked. I enjoyed shopping in the souks for furniture and crockery, making my new home comfortable and practical. I entertained the friends I'd made and enjoyed being single and free.

Most of my best memories from my happy Libyan days involve drinking sweet tea and eating the delicious food. The countryside was beautiful, filled with vineyards and orchards groaning with olives and fruit – and the most delicious peaches I ever tasted in my life. For the first time, I had regulated hours and days off. I could plan ahead and enjoy taking my mother out for drives in the country. Mum and I made a lot of wonderful friends among both the Libyans and international staff. We visited the Roman ruins and other archaeological sites like Leptis Magna, and Sabratha, an ancient Phoenician trading centre. Sometimes we drove to the beach or organized a '*wadi* bash' – a picnic and barbecue in a dry riverbed. We'd go in a convoy of cars and spend the whole day in the open air. When my sister was home on holiday, she joined us. These were some of the happiest days of my life.

Another first for me was cooking in my kitchen with my mother, which made us both surprisingly happy. We had so many fallen oranges and mandarins that we made jam and syrups and all manner of delights. It was the peaches, though, that really stick in my mind. On our drives through the vast plantations we'd stop and help ourselves to the huge juicy fruit. 'Let's find the farmstead and buy some to take home,' I told Mum one day. It took us ages to find and when we did, they laughed when we told them that we wanted to buy a dozen or so. 'We only sell by the truckload,' they replied. 'Open your boot and we'll fill it.' We went home with so many peaches that we had to give them away.

It was also in Libya that I saw gnarled old olive trees for the first time and learned how to harvest, soak and mature their fruit. Friends who had family groves gave us the fragrant green oil. As with a lot of Arab countries, there was always a bit of bartering and one of the most unusual bargains I ever struck was with an Italian dressmaker. One day she called by to drop something off for me and saw me picking snails from the orange trees before dropping them into a plastic bag. 'What are you going to do with those?' she asked.

'Throw them in the dustbin.'

'No, no, no!' she cried. '*Per favore*, you must give them to me! I will take all your snails. I make the most delicious soup from them. You must have some.' I never did take her up on her offer, but from that day on she received my snails and I had all my clothes made for free. I made some other wonderful friends in Tripoli, including a girl named Zanuba, the daughter of former African slaves who'd been owned by a wealthy Libyan family. Slaves weren't normally allowed an education, but she had gone to the Sudan to learn how to be a nurse and came back to work in the Mother and Child Health Services department under a British lady named Betty Sims, who was a technical adviser to the Ministry of Health. Zanuba invited Betty and me to meet her family, who were equally warm and generous. Her mother practically adopted me from day one, and frequently invited me to lunch to eat my favourite – grilled octopus on flatbread. They seemed proud that a woman of colour had done well enough to work for the United Nations and considered me a role model. When it was my birthday Zanuba told me that her mother was going to slaughter a sheep for me. 'What colour would you like?' she asked. When I looked puzzled, she added, 'Black, brown or white?'

'You choose,' I said, wondering what difference it would make. What I didn't realize was that three months later, I'd be presented with the fleece that her mother had tanned, dried and combed for me until it was the most beautiful soft white, brown and black fleeces hide. I used it as a rug, or a throw over my bed or on my sofa. I had six of them by the time I left Libya. Not surprisingly, I remained in contact with that wonderful family for more than twenty years.

Much as I was enjoying my new posting, my work there produced several challenges. One of the biggest was to convince parents to let their daughters become midwives. When we started, there were only a handful of Libyans on my staff. Zanuba was my best example, so she and I used to give talks in local schools to try to interest the girls and their families in joining our training programme. Just as in Somalia, basic education for girls was totally inadequate, so we had to spend a lot of time teaching them to read and speak English first. Once the girls got through the first six or so difficult months, they were able to do real midwifery with real patients. I'd go with them to the hospital and supervise their efforts to implement the practices we'd introduced in the classroom. Our training programme did a lot for Libya, and Libya did a lot for me. It was there that I was truly independent for the first time in my life, with my own money and my own career that wasn't dependent on my father or my husband. When I think about the state of that beautiful abundant country now, I could weep. Libya had been a Mediterranean paradise but two years after I left, its nationalist leader Colonel Gaddafi, who'd grown up as an impoverished goat herder, seized power in a military coup. Although he did much to modernize the country, improve literacy and keep the Islamic extremists under control, he was an eccentric and greedy dictator who also oppressed his people. Once Western forces ousted and killed him in 2011, the country fragmented into warring factions that have since further torn it apart.

Mohamed never stopped writing to me and I wrote back, but I was enjoying the freedom of my new life. I returned to Mogadishu a couple of times for short breaks but was secretly hoping to take up an offer of study leave after three years with the WHO, so that I could return to London and learn how to become a better trainer. I still loved Mohamed. I would always love him, but – as is often the case with Somali men – he had remarried his first wife and, deeply hurt, I didn't imagine that we would ever live together again.

After a year in Tripoli, I was allowed my first month-long annual leave and there was only one place I wanted to go – Djibouti. I withdrew $1,000 from my bank account, took a flight from Tripoli to Cairo to Aden to Djibouti and handed the money to my aunt Cecilia.

'What is this?' she asked, shocked.

'It is a small token of my thanks for all you did for me as a child,' I told her with a smile. My dear, hardworking, widowed auntie, who'd taken us waifs into her home and moulded us into the people we had become, was overwhelmed. With tears of pride and happiness in her eyes, she thanked me from the bottom of her heart. Within a decade, she would be dead from cancer, so I am grateful that I was able to repay some of her kindness while I could. I stayed in Djibouti for a while and reconnected with friends and family, but that too felt to have changed.

I wanted to visit Hargeisa so I flew to Aden only to discover that a strike meant no flights out for several days. I considered going by ship but there wasn't one for a week. I'd run out of money by then so the Somali embassy put me in a hotel near the airport to await the next flight. I arrived late and slept well as the hotel was surprisingly quiet. When I came down in the morning the place was empty and I asked a member of staff, 'Where is everyone?'

'You're our only guest,' he said. 'FLOSY has threatened to blow this hotel up.'

I contacted the embassy and told them I wanted to stay somewhere else, but they claimed there was nowhere else to go. 'Can't I sleep in the embassy?' They said it was already full with others seeking sanctuary. For the next four nights I barricaded myself into a rear room at the empty hotel and waited for a flight out, but none happened so I borrowed £20 from the embassy and persuaded them to buy me a ticket back to Djibouti, which I promised to refund. Once I was reunited with my aunt, she paid for me to travel on a truck driving to Somaliland.

I joined that overloaded truck for the 400-kilometre journey in the rainy season with my hair uncovered and wearing a summer top and short skirt. My suitcase was placed on top of the vehicle, which got stuck in the first riverbed. It was just like my school days. Everyone clambered out and I foolishly offered to help push only to be splattered with wet mud. We made it to the next village and became stuck again just as night was falling, so we decided to dig ourselves out in the morning. Everybody else was prepared and had sheets to wrap themselves in, but I had nothing. I was cold and wet and there were clouds of mosquitoes. The driver locked himself in his cabin alone. Thinking I was being smart, I walked to the riverbank and dug myself a grave in the wet mud and sand with my bare hands. I covered my feet and buried myself up to my neck to shelter from the bugs. In the morning I emerged from my tomb covered in the mud that caked my hair and face. A few of my fellow passengers saw me and were astonished. 'You slept there? Aren't you afraid of snakes?' Looking around nervously, I had to remind myself that I had survived. Wearily, I climbed back into the truck while they jacked it up, but somebody was injured in the process, so I had to climb down again to dress his wound, which added blood to the spatter pattern on my dress. I had no money left at all and by the time we arrived in Borama it was the middle of the night. Taking pity on me, the driver gave me a sheet stained with engine oil and sweat, and let me use his cabin. I woke at daybreak desperate to use the bathroom and – a Somali woman filthy from head to toe with a full bladder – I walked almost cross-legged to the customs booth to ask for help.

'Is there anywhere I can wash up? Is there water?' The customs officer looked me up and down disdainfully and shrugged. In a bitterly cold wind I walked to the hospital I knew well and approached the guard huddled at the gate. He looked at me as if I was deranged. 'Can I come in, please?' I asked.

'This place is a hospital,' he replied in a clipped tone. 'If you come in they will call the police, so you'd better go away.'

At that moment, I spotted a nurse in uniform and I pointed and said to him, 'See that nurse! Call her over. I want her!'...

He looked from me to her and said, 'You want Fatima?'

I nodded, through chattering teeth.

When the guard called the woman over I pulled myself to my full five feet two and a half inches and announced, 'I am *Ina Adan Dhakhtar.*'

She looked at me for a moment with a frown and then her eyes widened. 'Sister Edna?... You are not Edna!'

'Yes I am. We have just spent several days on the road. Please, can you help me get to a bathroom.'

She hesitated. 'Wait here.' I watched in dismay as she hurried back to the hospital and returned with a man from my clan who worked in the laboratory. 'This woman claims to be Edna Adan Ismail, your cousin. Do you know her?'

Thank goodness he recognized me immediately and cried, 'Edna! How are you?' He pulled the dirty sheet off me, instructed the guard to open the door and escorted me to his office. Within the hour I had used the bathroom, washed myself with soap and water, pulled a comb through my dirty hair and been given a clean sweater. He took me to his house where his wife cooked some food and gave me some clothes, perfume and make-up. I was so grateful to them both.

I had not a penny on me, but he arranged for a large official car to drive me to Hargeisa. Along the way we made a comfort stop for the driver, whereupon several poor people pressed around our vehicle to beg. I rolled down the window and told them, 'I'm so sorry, but I don't have any money.'

When the driver returned he shooed them away, telling them, 'Leave her be. This is the daughter of Adan Doctor!'

One old man shuffled off then and when he returned he knocked on the window and handed me a bowl of warm milk, just like the nectar I used to drink as a little girl. 'Milk for Adan Ismail's daughter,' he told me. 'Your father did so much for me. I owe him a lot, so please drink this. It is for you.'

I accepted the bowl with tears in my eyes. I think it was the most precious gift I ever received in my life. I drank some and passed the rest to a young woman near him whom I could see was breastfeeding. As we drove away, I blinked back the memories and thanked my father for still watching over me.

★★★

In July 1967, two months before I had completed my stint in Libya that would qualify me for a UK study leave, the recently elected President Abdirashid Ali Shermarke – in an attempt to unite the country – appointed my husband the Prime Minister of Somalia. It was a huge honour, especially for someone from Somaliland.

Mohamed wrote to me immediately. 'You have to come home, Edna. I need you here. Your country needs you. The UN can find somebody from out there in the big wide world to replace you… I can't.' Our correspondence resumed in earnest and I was reminded of his great skill with words. He had been invited on a diplomatic tour to America, London, Germany and Italy, he told me. At the height of the Cold War the West was keen to cement its relationship with those countries, like ours, who were strategically placed near the Suez Canal. This was even more important at a time when the Soviets were wooing the authorities in Mogadishu, generously providing huge quantities of military hardware and donating aid and other financial help to our struggling economy. They were also offering scholarships to all military officers (including my brother Farah) at training academies in Odessa and elsewhere. This was chiefly because although the British had trained all of Somaliland's Army officers to a high standard, they had all been removed from the army after 1961. This wasn't true of those from Italian Somalia. Before independence they had rarely risen above the rank of an NCO and were now being promoted beyond their experience or capability.

Mohamed assured me it would be considered 'scandalous' if the Prime Minister of the republic were to embark on this important world tour without his wife. He made for a convincing case. That summer he invited me to meet him on another shorter international trip he was taking so that we could discuss it further. I flew to the Grand Hotel in Rome and enjoyed probably the most romantic time I ever spent with the man I had married four years earlier. 'I love you, Edna,' he told me over a candlelit dinner. 'And I miss you. Let's not make the same mistake twice. We've both mellowed. I need you and you need me. We need each other. Our nation needs us both.'

I loved Mohamed, too. I had first fallen for him the night he danced with me in London and then sent me flowers the next day. I wanted to be with him as much as he wanted me by his side. I wasn't stupid; I knew that his desire to have me accompany him wasn't entirely personal. I was a trophy and an asset to his career – not just as a well-dressed employee of the UN who spoke several languages and knew how to behave in polite company but also as the daughter of Adan Doctor. To not be with him would reflect badly on us both. Still not quite convinced that

I wanted to be a First Lady as a full-time job, though, I went back to Libya to fulfil my commitments and think about my options, while Mohamed continued to bombard me with letters and long-distance telephone calls.

'Come home, Edna,' he'd plead. 'What do you say?' Although I'd be returning as his second wife, since his remarriage to the mother of his children, he assured me I would be the 'official' wife with all rights and privileges. By the time he finally wore me down and I decided to give him a second chance, I had only just signed a new contract to remain in Tripoli. My colleagues in Libya were shocked by my decision and refused to accept my resignation. 'You can't leave now, you've just got things going here!' they told me. The best they could do was persuade me to take one year's leave without pay, during which time I could reconsider my resignation. I'd keep my medical insurance and pension and in twelve months' time I could give them my final answer. It seemed like the best solution.

And so I returned to Mogadishu and to politics. There was no reason for me to go back other than my husband. My allegiance was not with Somalia but with Somaliland, and to a lesser extent the WHO. As I flew back to become the Prime Minister's consort I wondered what on earth I was letting myself in for.

CHAPTER TWELVE

Washington DC, USA, 1968

The presidential helicopter flew us to the West Lawn of the White House that blustery mid-March day in 1968. We'd been collected from Andrews Air Force Base on the start of our week-long American tour and landed on the West Lawn from where a limousine drove us the short distance to where we were to be met by the President of the United States. I had been back with my husband for less than three months and yet my feet had hardly touched the ground.

President Lyndon Johnson and his wife 'Lady Bird' were waiting to greet us in the chill morning breeze, as a twenty-one-gun salute was sounded as our limousine – bearing the twin flags of the US and Somalia – brought us to a halt. Smoothing down the lemon yellow dress and matching coat I'd bought in Rome especially, I held onto my fur hat as I was assisted out of the limo and took my place beside my husband as he shook hands with the man who'd stepped in after John F. Kennedy's assassination five years earlier. I was thirty years old and the new President was twice my age. 'Welcome to Washington, Mrs Egal,' he said, smiling warmly to put me immediately at ease. Mohamed and I had no idea that, within weeks, the man known affectionately as 'LBJ' would shock the nation by announcing his decision not to seek a second term. Lady Bird was polite but far cooler towards me, so I was relieved to be presented to Virginia Rusk, the wife of Secretary of State Dean Rusk, and Muriel Humphrey, the wife of the Vice President, Hubert Humphrey. Both ladies were instantly kind and maternal towards me, the 'young girl' in their midst.

I was also assigned a lady-in-waiting of sorts. A woman named Evelyn Symington, the wife of a senator, took care of me and guided me through the minefield of diplomatic protocol. For example, nobody had told me that if I was ever presented with flowers at a public event it was best to pass them to an aide so that I could continue to shake hands. Our day had started so early with a 4 a.m. hairdressing appointment for me in our suite at the Waldorf Astoria Hotel in Manhattan, then a 6 a.m. flight to DC. On the lawn of the White House, Lady Bird Johnson handed me a bouquet of roses, which I then held onto throughout the entire meet and greet ceremony before being escorted to the South Lawn for a press conference.

As camera shutters clicked and TV cameras rolled, I clung to my bouquet like a deflating lifebelt as the President addressed Mohamed publicly. He said, 'We have watched with interest and admiration the development of the Somali Republic in the last eight years. We know that you have succeeded in building one of the most effective democratic governments in all of Africa. We are aware of your noble efforts to bury ancient antagonisms and to get on with the work of peace… I had hoped that we might welcome you this morning in the warm glow of a Washington spring, but Mother Nature has seen fit to give us instead just a parting taste of winter. But I know that you will find that our friendship for you and for your people flourishes in every season. Mr Prime Minister, we bid you and your lovely lady the warmest of our welcomes.'

After further introductions and handshaking, it was Mrs Rusk who saved the day – and the flowers – when she asked me, 'Would you like me to take these from you, dear? You might find it easier.' Unless she had kindly intervened, I'd have gone through the whole day carrying that bouquet. So you see, I was not quite ready for the diplomatic life.

Our next few days in the American capital were a dizzying round of engagements as Mohamed held intense discussions with the worried Americans about the increasing Russian interest in the Horn of Africa. As was the way of things, I wasn't included in these talks and was taken instead to visit a hospital and a school where children and adults lined the streets and performed for us. Sometimes I was asked to make speeches, but I hadn't been prepared for that and had no idea what to say.

These were the kinds of things I gradually learned to do better as time went on. With experience, I improved at improvising. But new to this kind of life and with a camera or microphone in my face, I didn't find public speaking easy. When I was reunited with Mohamed in our hotel I would often take out my frustration on him but he'd just laugh and say, 'Talk to them about nursing, if you can't think of anything else.' It was the nature of our relationship that I took that as an insult, belittling nursing, as if that was the only thing I could talk about. We would then snap at each other all night, before having to smile for the cameras the next day. Travelling as a First Lady was not always a bouquet of roses.

The one thing I was grateful to Mohamed for, however, was the $10,000 budget he had given me to buy clothes for my new role. Having grown up in a wealthy family, money meant nothing to him and everything had a price. He often showered me with extravagant gifts, bringing me back a Christian Dior gold cigarette case and matching lighter or six designer handbags from Europe. He showed the kind of generosity that most wives would have appreciated but, unfortunately for Mohamed, the daughter of Adan Doctor considered such expenditure wasteful and his gestures weren't always appreciated.

I remember one time I happened to comment that the wife of the Indian ambassador was wearing the most beautiful sari I had ever seen, which she wore so elegantly. Before I knew it, Mohamed, while on a diplomatic visit in Nairobi, had one of his aides go to the Indian quarter and buy me twelve of the most expensive silk saris he could find. One sari would have been a thoughtful gesture but twelve was obscene and I told him so. That sparked a row that lasted for days. 'A silk scarf or a bottle of perfume would have sufficed,' I told him. 'Something simple to let me know that you thought of me. You should know by now that gestures are far more valuable to me than gifts.'

When it came to the budget he gave me for our forthcoming world tour, however, I didn't complain. First I met with the wife of the US embassy's *chargé d'affaires* in Mogadishu, who advised me on my itinerary and suggested we buy raincoats and be prepared for the cooler climate. Then I flew to Rome in the company of a beautiful Italian named Maria Louisa Bonanni, known as Marilou, the press agent for the Prime Minister's office. With Marilou by my side in Rome I chose the tailored lemon dress and white long coat that reminded me of the elegance of Jackie Kennedy. We then selected matching shoes, gloves and a handbag. Her instructions were to make sure I looked the part, which I thought rather ridiculous at first as I felt perfectly capable of deciding what to wear and when – if it was even noticed. A few weeks earlier I'd dressed up for the state visit of President Kenneth Kaunda of Zambia only to be introduced to him just the once with a brief handshake and a smile and then cast aside as superfluous to requirements. I'd expected to have far more involvement as the Prime Minister's wife, but I hadn't yet fully appreciated how much men dominated these events. Indignant, I mused that I could have stayed on a little longer in Libya and continued with my valuable work.

Neither Mohamed nor I had ever been to America before, so we were very excited about the trip. When we arrived we were accommodated in the historic Blair House, the President's Guest House on Pennsylvania Avenue, where I was presented with a 'wardrobe assistant' who asked, 'Do you need help dressing?' and, 'Is there anything you would like to have ironed?' I am certain I offended her when I told her that I could do my own ironing because she kept saying, 'But Madam, I can do that for you.' Later that night we were the guests at a glittering gala dinner at the White House and the following evening at a reception at the Somali embassy in Washington. Instead of putting on one of my expensive Italian cocktail dresses, I chose to wear a *guntiino,* a Somali traditional dress worn almost like a sari in a colourful print bought for about 100 shillings (£15) from a *suuq* or market in Mogadishu. It felt right for the occasion and everyone commented on the appropriateness of my attire. The following day, we were flown in Air Force One from Washington to the Tennessee Valley Authority to visit the vast Wilson Dam, where its engineers assured our delegation that they had the expertise and the funding to build similar projects anywhere in the world. Then we were flown on to Cape Canaveral in Florida to see the Kennedy Space Center. We had a tour of the *Apollo 11* rocket that would land the first man on the moon the following year, and signed its logbook that went into space.

For the most part, people went out of their way to make us feel very welcome and comfortable. However, I do recall one unpleasant episode during our visit that affected members of our delegation. A few of them hoped to experience the nightlife

on Coco Beach after our visit to the space centre and went out
unaccompanied that night. They stopped at a restaurant, but were
refused service because of the colour of their skin. They came
back to the hotel and let everyone know that segregation was
still alive and well in the US, or at least in that part of Florida.
I remember being so shocked by that. We knew about apartheid
in South Africa, of course, and I'd attended rallies against it in
Hyde Park when I was a student in London, but America felt so
liberal and different. I had my eyes truly opened there when one
of our aides explained the issues behind the rise of the American
civil rights movement.

White supremacists apart, the Americans saw Mohamed as
a friend of the West – a well-spoken, pro-democracy African
political leader who supported their interests, and they were
keen to woo him and gain his allegiance. None more so than the
President, who at the state banquet on our final night, delivered
a most embracing speech. 'We are all egalitarians tonight, not
only in our belief in the equality of man, but in our admiration
of a man for whom that philosophy might have been named,' he
began. 'No statesman is struggling harder today to realize the
dream of democracy for his own people than the man that we
honour tonight, Prime Minister Egal.'

Turning to Mohamed, he added, 'Your words have always
served the cause of peace. You have stayed the arrows of conflict,
which threatened to bring bloodshed to the Horn of Africa.
And you have lost no time and neglected no opportunity in the
search for true progress for all of your people. You come to us
from a new Africa where change is as certain as the sunrise. You
are one of those who have determined that change shall always
mean promise for your people. You have helped to found a true
democracy, where each man has a voice in his nation's future.

You have done much to lessen the tensions that threatened East Africa with the waste of war. And you have begun the long, hard job of economic development to bring your people the food and shelter and education that all men seek and that all men deserve... We here in the United States are inspired by your courage. We admire your perseverance. And most of all we are delighted by your presence here this evening. Ladies and gentlemen, I invite you to join me now in a toast to a wise leader and his people. To the President and to the people of the Somali Republic – and to the Prime Minister and his charming lady, Mrs Egal.'

I don't think I had ever been prouder of Mohamed than I was that night. Our relationship was unique, some might say tumultuous, but even when we were angry at each other there remained a reservoir of deep mutual respect. He used to tell me, 'Edna, you are as close an intellectual match as I can find in Somaliland.' Even when he was in charge of our country he would often ask me to vet his most important speeches, policy proposals, or political communiqués from the Prime Minister's office. I didn't know shorthand so I'd take down his words in longhand, get his secretary to type them up, make corrections and pass them back. When we were travelling I'd jot down ideas on anything from a dinner napkin to toilet paper, slipping the notes into my pocket for the two of us to discuss later.

I know that he was proud of me and never more so than at the White House. Sitting next to the President in my yellow silk dress covered in sequins and matching shoes, LBJ and I chatted easily, finding common ground in our love of food. As he passed me some chutney, we shared our passion for chillies, peppers and spices. He was so gallant and good at putting people at their ease. He asked me about my nursing career and my training in London and was surprised that I planned to carry on working in a Mogadishu hospital. 'My husband and his aides hate that I want to,' I confided. 'It is unheard of and unthinkable in my country. They keep telling Mohamed that having a wife who works will lose him votes, but then I've never been a conventional First Lady. To begin with, I'm far too thin.'

'Really?' LBJ asked, amazed.

'Yes, Mr President. The wife of a Prime Minister of Somalia is expected to be fat because to be fat is to be wealthy, as well as being a sign of maturity and therefore wisdom.' We laughed together at that, and got along very well for the rest of the evening – so much so that Mohamed joked afterwards that perhaps he should be worried about what the President and I were laughing about. It was his way of telling me that I had done well. At the end of the dinner, the President signed the official menu for me and then the White House catering staff surprised me with a white chocolate 'Mousse Shukri' made in my honour, which almost made me cry. If only I could have told my father about that most memorable of nights.

★★★

From Florida we flew to New York where Mohamed addressed the United Nations for the first time. I was far more excited about walking into that 'Temple of the World' than almost anything else we'd done. I gazed in awe at all the different nations' flags and paintings, the national treasures and trophies, and was honoured to meet U Thant, the Secretary-General. Being there felt very special, and I still feel that way each time I visit the UN.

Probably our nicest experience of our entire US trip was taking the evening off from our ever-present bodyguards to visit Times Square one night. We found a little Italian restaurant and sat in a corner to enjoy a steak and spaghetti dinner. That felt like the first time that we'd had any privacy and weren't surrounded by people telling us what to do and where to go. For that evening only, we felt like a normal couple on holiday, although we later learned that security servicemen and women in plain clothes were watching us all the time.

From New York we flew to London, where we were given a suite at the Dorchester Hotel in Park Lane. At our lunch with Prime Minister Harold Wilson, the Foreign Secretary and the Secretary of Health I made another faux pas. I smoked cigarettes in those days and after dessert, I pulled out the flashy gold case Mohamed had bought me and selected a cigarette. The Minister of Health leaned towards me and said, quietly, 'I'd be happy to light that for you after we have toasted her Majesty.' The protocol hadn't been explained to me and I felt such a fool.

I received gifts from President Charles De Gaulle during Mohamed's state visit to France and in West Germany we were the guests of Chancellor Kiesinger. In Rome I made my next mistake by going shopping instead of meeting Mohamed for a diplomatic lunch with the Italian Foreign Minister Amintore Fanfani, the man who'd been Prime Minister during Somalia's early independence years. His aides found me browsing in a store and hurried me to the villa, where I sheepishly joined the meal halfway through. On our final night when all the meetings were over, Mohamed and I went to a nightclub and danced to 'I Left My Heart in San Francisco' by Tony Bennett, a song whose lyrics seemed so appropriate before we went home to our own city by the bay. It was a romantic end to our tour and I was so proud of what my husband had achieved, but I think I knew even then that this life wasn't for me. I was still so young and couldn't help thinking that the political world was made up of people far older than me. I wasn't prepared for state visits and meeting with presidents. I hadn't been trained. I didn't like pomp and ceremony, and I didn't want to be in the political limelight. I was simply the daughter of Adan Doctor.

I was simply a midwife.

★★★

Back home in Mogadishu, Mohamed and I settled back into the life we'd made for ourselves there. Our new home was the Prime Minister's official residence in the exclusive Lido area where most of the foreign diplomats and consultants rented houses. Mohamed had it redecorated by an Italian interior designer in a very lavish and extravagant style with the kind of fussy and overbearing furniture that I hated. I was never consulted – he did it to surprise me and was disappointed when I said how much I hated it.

It was no coincidence that Russian 'diplomats' moved into the next property. They were really KGB agents so we had to cope with their increasing scrutiny. Mohamed warned me from the outset that our home was bugged and that if we wanted to discuss anything personal, we should go to the verandah on the other side of the house. Cold War politics was beginning to affect even us. He was, after all, the blue-eyed boy as far as the West was concerned, and it didn't help that we had just returned from this successful trip to America and other capitalist countries.

Hassan Kayd, my childhood friend and the leader of the 1961 coup, had returned from the UN in New York by then and was working in Mogadishu as a security consultant. Mohamed thought that Hassan's military background and his longstanding connections to me for having saved his life meant he was ideal to check out our household security system in light of our new neighbours.

Hassan agreed and at some point the next day, he returned unannounced, sneaked over the wall surrounding our compound, entered the house, and stole one of my husband's scarves from the bedroom. When he brought it to us the following day and explained how easy it had been for him to break in, we knew we needed a security upgrade. Thanks to him, the compound wall was raised, broken glass was cemented into its ridge and Hassan replaced our guard detail with men he knew and trusted.

It isn't easy to be the wife of a politician, and once I became the 'First Lady' a great deal more was expected of me, with endless obligations. In addition to all the ceremonial activities, there were campaigns and local elections, for which I toured the country, sometimes with my husband and sometimes alone, to try to convince people to support Mohamed under President Shermarke. Despite our differences, I always felt I was campaigning for the best politician the Somali people ever had, a conviction I have to this day. We were also constantly receiving diplomats, dignitaries from abroad, local politicians and men of influence. One of the guests I resented the most, and who arrived promptly at nine o'clock every night to brief Mohamed on the day's events, was the Commander-in-Chief of the Somali Army, Major General Mohamed Siad Barre. He was twenty years older than me, tall and with a strange fuzz of a moustache that gave him the appearance of Adolf Hitler. He spoke loudly and deeply and held an authoritarian and regimental demeanour. I gave him the nickname 'General Boots' because he wore military boots so thickly spread with boot polish that it was like jam. Each time he walked into my lounge, which had a cream carpet and beige sofas, he would leave annoying brown stains, especially when he sat fidgeting and shuffling his feet while talking. I complained to Mohamed, 'At least try to see to it that General Boots sits in the same chair because he's staining a different seat every time he calls!' Barre's other annoying habit was that when he smoked he disrespectfully flicked his ash on the carpet rather than in any of the ashtrays provided. He used matches and when they were spent he'd chew on them and spit splinters of matchwood all over my carpet, too.

Born in the Ogaden region of the Ethiopian empire, Siad Barre had risen through the ranks to a position of power with a strong sense of Somali nationalism. He had also become a staunch advocate of socialism after training in the Soviet Union. Mohamed didn't like or trust him either, but we both knew that we had to be civil regardless. In my quest to be a better political wife, I decided to invite him to a social event at our home one night – in spite of his boots. We would sometimes borrow American movies from the United States Information Service Library and screen them in our compound, asking friends and colleagues from the foreign diplomatic corps to join us. I was particularly fond of the French ambassador's wife who was a frequent visitor. I once asked Barre to join us for *Dr Zhivago* but my husband was not pleased. After he'd left, Mohamed said, 'I hope your inclusion of that nincompoop in our gathering doesn't put any ideas in his head. I fear he is an ambitious man.'

How ambitious we would soon learn.

★★★

Whenever I wasn't tied up with diplomatic or other commitments, I put on my plain white nurse's uniform, tied my hair in a chignon, and went to work two days a week in the maternity ward at the Digfer general hospital in Mogadishu. I looked like every other nurse in the hospital, except that my clothes were cleaned and pressed twice a week.

Not surprisingly perhaps, many people thought that delivering babies and supervising nursing students was inappropriate for a First Lady. 'How can the Prime Minister's wife be working in a hospital?' they'd ask. 'This is shameful and undignified; it is a political embarrassment to Egal and to the Party.' I thought that people would have known by then that nursing was my real vocation. Whose daughter was I, after all? Politics was a burden, something I had to bear for the sake of my husband and, I suppose, for the sake of my country. At first Mohamed tried to talk me out of it, but I think he knew in his heart the kind of woman he was married to. Ignoring his objections, I'd arrive at the hospital in my crisp uniform at 7 a.m. sharp even though I had no clock to punch because I wanted to teach my students the value of punctuality. Like my father before me, I urged them to treat people with dignity regardless of how poor or uneducated they were. I wanted to show them that if the wife of a Prime Minister could speak with respect to a patient, be punctual, listen, and actuality 'hear' what the patient was trying to say, then they could certainly do the same. It was a matter of setting standards for future health professionals, a golden opportunity that I was not going to allow to pass me by.

The Italians built Digfer Hospital in the 1960s, and whoever constructed it had clearly never worked in a hospital and certainly not in a developing country. To start with it had four floors, instead of easily accessible ground floor pavilions like most of the others. Badly maintained from the start, the lifts failed in the first few months, which meant everyone had to climb or be carried up the stairs. The operating area was accessible from all sides, like the Arc de Triomphe, which meant that it couldn't be kept sterile. The wards were long and gloomy and when the doors were shut the corridors so dark that you had to turn the lights on – if the electricity was working.

Being the wife of the PM did have some advantages in that it allowed me to accomplish some things for the hospital that might not have been possible otherwise. Because of my position, I persuaded the government to pay for the walls to be painted and necessary repairs to be made. We refurbished the entire maternity ward and were given new sheets for the beds and new uniforms for the staff. I knew that my old hospital in Hargeisa and many others across our land were equally in need but my plan was to fix Digfer and show them what could be done before I began on the rest. I also contacted Miss Markham, my former nurse tutor at West London Hospital, and started to make the arrangements to bring her to Somalia. She had been a great teacher, so I invited her to come as a consultant and advise me on the training of midwives. To my surprise and delight she agreed, so we set about fixing a date for the end of 1969 when she would become available. I couldn't wait to see her again and benefit from her expertise.

My biggest challenge at Digfer was to rid the hospital of its plague of bedbugs. First we tried fumigating the beds and using insecticides, but that didn't do any good. The entire maternity ward was badly infested. The only thing that worked was to wheel the metal beds outside and, using a blowtorch, run its flame around the entire frame until the bugs burst and burned. Then we'd scrape and sand the frames before repainting them.

Mohamed hated me doing this work most of all. 'It isn't right, Edna!' he told me, exasperated, when he asked about my day. 'What if someone sees the wife of a Prime Minister in the hospital courtyard killing bugs with blowtorches? Think of the embarrassment!' One look from me told him that he had no choice other than to hope the news didn't get out. The best he could get from me was a reassurance that I wouldn't bring bedbugs home from work with me.

One of the things that caused me great irritation was the government's insistence that I have a bodyguard, which seemed ridiculous as I wasn't the kind of person people wanted to kill and was certainly not easy to follow around. Even today, colleagues complain that I rush around everywhere, making random stops to talk to patients or chat with their relatives. I am hard to pin down. When out driving, I often stop to give strangers a ride or spontaneously accept a lift from an acquaintance. How was a bodyguard going to keep up? Ignoring my objections, the authorities assigned me a tall, tough-looking man who knew little about health and nothing at all about maternity wards. In spite of this, he had instructions to follow me wherever I went. I complained to that poor man every day. 'Who are you trying to protect me from? Newborn babies? Women in labour? My students? And, no, you can't come into the delivery room. It is forbidden.'

Eventually he resigned himself to sitting outside the door of the delivery room. As soon as I emerged to rush to another ward, he'd jump up to follow me, stopping only when I reminded him, 'No, no, no, I am still inside the hospital, remember? You don't follow me in the hospital. Period.'

I gave him a hard time, not because of anything he had done but because I was angry by the mere idea of him following me around. Nothing in my experience allowed me to believe that we lived in the kind of country where politicians and their wives might be kidnapped or killed. I knew that other African politicians had been assassinated in recent years, including three prime ministers from Burundi, three cabinet ministers from the Congo, the prime minister of Ethiopia, and two Kenyan ministers, but nothing like that had ever happened in Somaliland or Somalia at that time and I didn't believe it ever would.

Or so I thought.

CHAPTER THIRTEEN

London, England, 1969

On 15 October 1969, I was resting in my hotel room in London after yet another day of fertility tests at St Thomas' Hospital where around ten years earlier I had taken my final exams as a student nurse. In spite of our frequent disagreements, Mohamed and I never stopped wanting a child together, but at the age of thirty-two and after six years of trying it seemed increasingly likely that it was impossible for me. The thought of never being delivered of my own baby almost broke my heart.

A frantic banging on the door woke me from my nap and I opened it to find Marilou Bonanni, my aide and friend, distraught in the corridor. 'Oh, Edna, *mia poverina!*' she cried, waving her hands expressively and jumbling Italian and English. Coming into the room in a fluster, she looked at me wide-eyed and blurted, 'I just heard it on the BBC news. The President has been assassinated!'

Winded, I sat down hard on the bed and asked her to repeat what she had just said. 'President Shermarke is dead. He was shot by his bodyguard on an official visit to the town of Las Anod,' she told me. 'My press contacts just confirmed it.'

I held my head in my hands and burst into tears. I couldn't believe what she was telling me. Shermarke was a good man and the President who'd appointed my husband despite opposition, and he had been trying to steer our country through the labyrinth of post-colonial rule. I'd only met him once or twice, but he was my husband's political ally and I knew his death would create a dangerous vacuum. When I finally caught my breath, I telephoned the Somali embassy in London to ask them for news. To my astonishment, they said they'd known for a few hours but didn't know how to break it to me. They added that Somali radio was only broadcasting prayers from the Qur'an.

'Has my husband been informed?' I asked. The reply came that they were still trying to reach him. Checking my watch, I estimated that Mohamed would have recently arrived in California, having been invited there after once again addressing the UN in New York. He was planning on staying with his old friend William Holden in Los Angeles before returning to London to join me.

There was no question about who I'd call next – Colonel Crook, my friend and mentor, long retired from the Colonial Office. I visited him every time I was in London and had seen him just a few days earlier. I knew that he would be able to find out more information for me through his intelligence contacts. I was right. 'Stay where you are and don't talk to anyone,' he instructed on the telephone, after confirming that our President was dead. 'I'll be right over.' That lovely old man with his handlebar moustache came straight to my hotel in Lancaster Gate from his home by the river in Surrey and offered to help me in any way he could. The kind colonel brought a doctor friend of mine with him in case I needed any medical attention following the shocking news.

With his usual efficiency, Colonel Crook spoke to the hotel manager and arranged for Marilou to be moved to the adjoining room, all the while assuring me that the assassination was an isolated incident and that I had nothing to fear. Both of us kept calling the embassy for further news and eventually heard that Mohamed was in transit and would meet me at Heathrow airport the following morning. 'He will then fly back to Mogadishu to arrange the funeral and begin the process for the appointment of a new President,' I was told.

'Then I will be by his side,' I replied. For once in my married life, I knew exactly where I had to be. Several hours later I found myself with my suitcase waiting for my husband in the VIP lounge at the airport watching his plane taxi to a halt. My understanding was that there wouldn't be much time before we had to board our Alitalia flight to Rome, Addis Ababa and finally to Mogadishu, where I knew my mother, brother and sister would be anxiously waiting. When he finally walked into the lounge, Mohamed looked five years older and it had nothing to do with his eleven-hour flight. His jaw was set and his expression grim. We embraced and I whispered, 'Are you all right?' He nodded briskly before turning to his diplomats to discuss last-minute arrangements.

After a few minutes he turned back to me and, taking my shoulders in his hands, he stared deep into my eyes. 'Edna, you are not to come home with me,' he said firmly.

I shook my head and began to protest. 'No! Why not? What about you?'

'I have to go back. There is much to do and I am head of the government.'

'But...'

He silenced me with a look. 'None of us know what will happen next, Edna... One never knows when there is political turmoil in Africa. You have to stay here where I know you're safe and then I will send for you... okay?'

There was no arguing with him, so I brushed away my tears and nodded. He had further instructions for me. 'You must move from the hotel immediately. I've made arrangements for you to stay with friends in West London. They'll be happy to have you.'

'Don't tell anyone where you are going and don't call anyone but Colonel Crook,' he added.

'Am I in danger?' I asked.

'I don't know.'

'Are you?'

'Don't worry about me. Siad Barre and the Somali Army will protect me. I just need to go home and find out which clan is behind this assassination, and who might be next.' He handed me some cash to take care of any personal expenses and arranged that the embassy cover my hotel bill and provide me with a car and driver. His final request was that I keep an eye on his daughter Amina who was studying in London, and two of his sons, Ali and Ahmed, who were at school in Switzerland. 'Tell them to lie low.'

Trying not to cry, I kissed Mohamed goodbye and watched him walk away, not knowing if I would ever see him again.

★★★

In a daze I was driven back to the hotel where I waited for Colonel Crook to escort me to the safe house – somewhere that even the embassy wouldn't be able to find me. He arrived with the news that he'd been assured the British would offer me political asylum if I wished to remain in the UK indefinitely.

'Thank you, but no,' I told him. 'I will join my husband as soon as I can.'

Mr and Mrs Holland, a retired couple in their seventies who had been Mohamed's landlords when he was a student in London, were welcoming and kind and I did my best to settle into their house in Chiswick, west London, where they lived modestly as retired schoolteachers. Bless her, Mrs Holland even bought satin sheets for my bed, assuming that a Prime Minister's wife would sleep on nothing less. For the next few days I hardly went out and waited in hoping to hear from Mohamed, but he never called. I told myself he was undoubtedly very busy. I heard from Colonel Crook and others that the preparations for the President's state funeral were going as planned, with regional and international heads of state flying in. A nighttime curfew had been imposed to avoid any demonstrations and the atmosphere was tense. I felt so helpless in London and only wished I could be by Mohamed's side.

Then on 21 October, one day after the funeral, there was more shocking news: there had been a military coup in Somalia. The reports said the Army had taken over to 'prevent civilian unrest'. Colonel Crook informed me that all members of parliament had been taken to a safe place for their protection. The truth, when I discovered it much later, was far more chilling. At 3 a.m. soldiers acting on the orders of senior officers had woken Mohamed and his ministers from their homes, ordered them to dress, and driven them thirty kilometres beyond Mogadishu to the fortified country home of the President in a rural town called Afgoi, where they were placed under house arrest. The rest of the parliament had also been sent there, and anyone else who was suspected of creating trouble was arrested.

For twenty-four terrible hours, no one could tell me what had happened to Mohamed and the rest of his government. Nor did I know if my mother, brother and sister were safe, as I imagined fighting on the streets and all kinds of horrors. The first I knew that the change of power was official was when the Somali Embassy in London refused to take my calls and stopped offering me a car and driver. They cut me off. I was left without any diplomatic status or access to intelligence and felt helpless and afraid. Frustrated, I called Colonel Crook and told him, 'I need to go home.' He did his best to dissuade me, as did my hosts who kindly told me, 'You can stay here as long as you like', but my mind was set.

'Thank you but no,' I said. 'My family, my home, and my animals are in Mogadishu. I only have $83 left to my name but I still have my return ticket. I need to get back and do whatever needs to be done. I would rather take my chances there than sit here and do nothing.'

It wasn't until the third or the fourth day that we had confirmation that the leader of the coup was 'General Boots' himself, Major-General Siad Barre, supported by some thirty senior officers and the Soviet advisers who'd been grooming him for years. Barre had crowned himself not President at first, but Chairman of the Supreme Revolutionary Council (the title of 'President' would come later), creating the kind of socialist junta the Americans and British had feared. My usually clever husband, who'd believed Barre would protect him, had flown straight into a trap.

Thankfully, my airline ticket was still valid, so I sent a telegram to my brother to tell him which flight I'd be arriving on. It was only when I arrived at Mogadishu airport three weeks after the coup to be met by senior members of the security police that I realized that Farah never even received my note. 'Welcome home, Mrs Egal,' said the smiling men in suits and sunglasses. They would soon become part of Siad Barre's feared National Security Service or NSS, trained by the KGB. They ushered me quickly into a waiting car and as we drove out of the airport the driver turned left instead of right, so I asked, 'Where are you taking me?'

'Don't you want to say hello to your mother?'

'Well, yes, of course.'

My relatives had no idea that I was home, and were very emotional to see me. Farah and Asha and my mother all embraced me and we wept together at the sorrow of our situation. Almost as soon as I crossed the threshold, the security police took away my passport and told me that I was under total house arrest. I was not permitted to leave the building otherwise I would be taken to prison. They added that anyone leaving or visiting me would be stopped and searched by the security police who would be stationed outside night and day. When I began to protest that I needed to go home to see to my animals and pick up clothes and other belongings, the men stopped smiling.

'We are being respectful to you, Mrs Egal,' they told me, coldly. 'Don't give us any trouble. Your home, cars and property belong to the government now.' Exhausted and emotionally drained, I didn't have the energy to argue and only wanted them to get out of our three-bedroom house I had bought for my family after we returned from Libya. Collapsing into an armchair, I caught up with all their news and the shocking realization that I too had walked straight into Siad Barre's trap.

My chief concern was for Mohamed, so I started to write the first of many letters to him, explaining that I was back in the country to campaign for his release. I asked if there was anything he needed, suspecting he probably only had the clothes he was arrested in. I never knew if he received the letters I asked the security police to deliver, and I received nothing back.

Farah was married and my sister Asha had recently become engaged to a friend of his and moved in with my mother until her wedding. She and my mother were allowed to leave the house for work, basic errands, food shopping and to buy jerrycans of water.

With no money of my own and my bank account emptied of the
$20,000 I'd saved while working for the WHO, we had no choice
but to live on my brother's salary as an Army officer. Mercifully,
he was still being paid. I was also happy at least that Asha was
somewhere I could keep an eye on her, or I might never have
been able to see her. I was also grateful for the clothes she lent me,
as I had only what little was in my suitcase for a European trip,
which was totally inappropriate for Somalia. Every day I told the
police that I had to be allowed to return to my house, but they
ignored my requests. I'd heard through the grapevine that our
beautiful home in the Lido had been turned into something Barre
and his men dubbed 'Edna's nightclub'. Fearful for my beloved
cheetah Sanu, I made some calls and pulled some strings and was
finally permitted to go home under armed escort to pick up some
of my personal things.

The sight that greeted me there was truly horrible. The house
was unrecognizable, littered with empty bottles, overflowing
ashtrays and stains all over the carpets and furniture. There was
half-eaten food and dirty plates everywhere. Our personal items
such as valuable cigarette cases, lighters and a gold dagger were
missing, no doubt given as gifts to the families of the thieving
officers, and our safe was swinging open with all its contents
missing. Aside from irreplaceable personal documents, photographs and my father's letters to me in London, I'd also lost all
my remaining jewellery and that of my mother, which – ironically – I'd persuaded her to let me keep for safety. Our home felt
contaminated and abused.

I almost wept when I saw Sanu, who was still alive and in his
cage but was thin, dirty and extremely fearful. Pulling myself
together I was determined not to let the soldiers see me cry and
begged the police to allow me to take my baby. 'He needs to be

with me,' I told them. 'Please, you can have everything else that I possess, just let me take my cheetah home.'

'No. He belongs to the government now.'

'But I raised him! He's like my baby!' I fought to remain calm. No matter how much I pleaded, they refused to let me take him and hurried me out of the house with just a suitcase full of clothes. It was not long afterwards that I heard that my dear Sanu had been shot dead after the soldiers claimed he'd been aggressive towards them. Sanu could never attack anybody. I was sure they killed him for his fur. My heart felt truly broken.

For the next six months I remained trapped at my mother's house, unable to leave, see any of my friends or even go to the market. There was still no word from Mohamed and I felt ever more helpless. Suffocating, I would have been happier if they had sentenced me to hard labour breaking up rocks or tilling the land than being stuck inside day and night. This was the worst punishment they could give me. I longed to walk free in the bush with the camels or visit the lush hills of Borama. I wished I could paddle in the waters of the Indian Ocean where once we went lobster fishing at low tide during the full moon, or just see more than the small patch of sky above our compound. If anyone called to visit – and few were brave enough to – they were treated roughly and searched thoroughly to make sure that they weren't carrying messages or that I wasn't giving them things to take away. Every now and then the security police would burst in uninvited and ransack our home, searching the toilet tanks, opening cupboards and drawers and examining everything from food to the insides of packets of cigarettes, which I was smoking again out of stress.

The national radio station and newspapers had been taken over by the authorities, so we had limited access to real news. Foreign broadcasts were banned but we were able to listen to the BBC

Somali Service on shortwave radio if we could buy batteries, although after Somalia destroyed the BBC relay station in Berbera the service was terrible. Mainly though, we heard whatever the regime wanted us to hear – chiefly our new 'leader' in his booming voice blaring out plans for our new nation under what he called 'scientific socialism'. Barre, who'd become known as *Afweyne* or 'Big Mouth', came up with his unique political ideology because he couldn't call us Communists as they are atheists and that would have alienated all Muslims. Instead, he developed a kind of 'pick and mix' policy combining Marxism and the teachings of the Qur'an. Regimental discipline was brought into every aspect of our lives and there was no freedom of speech or movement, no free press and no political parties.

The new regime allowed him to become a dictator. All capitalists were labelled 'Imperialist pigs' and hundreds more people were arrested. Capitalism was bad for everyone except for Barre and his friends who were handsomely rewarded with property, contracts and trade. Clan names were abandoned and so, in theory, was our allegiance to them. We were all now to be addressed as *jaale,* which means 'comrade' and expected to adapt immediately to the new politics decreed by his politburo.

As the tension ramped up, armed men in uniform would arrive late at night, sending my mother into a blind panic. They'd push us into one room while they once again searched our house, ripping open cushions and mattresses with knives, overturning furniture and casting much loved records from their sleeves. This kind of brutality was being repeated all over the country and much worse – sons were taken and women raped if they didn't hand over jewellery or cash. Or even if they did. Furious at the way we and others were being treated, I greeted our intruders with nothing but contempt. On one late night search of our home, I asked them, 'Are you sure you don't want to check out the helicopter on my roof?' To my astonishment, one of them climbed up to take a look. The only way I could get my own back on them was to have them see my smiling face as they left our house.

My house arrest came to an unexpected end thanks to my nursing skills and the misfortune of others. One day Radio Mogadishu broadcast an urgent appeal for blood donors and for anyone with nursing skills. There had been a fire at the prestigious Juba Hotel and many people were injured. As soon as I heard this, I knew that I had to help, so I put on my white coat and prepared to walk to the hospital.

'What are you doing, Edna?' my mother cried, with an expression of horror.

'Going to look after the injured at the hospital' I said. Shrugging, I added, 'What will they do to me, Mum? Shoot me?' In my heart I knew that was a possibility so, taking my courage in both hands, I walked out of the house and confronted the surprised guards. 'I'm needed urgently at Digfer Hospital,' I told them. 'They want help with the victims of the fire and you know I can help. You can either follow me or wait until I return home.' Then I started walking. They followed me for a while and then dropped back, presumably to report my insubordination.

I found the hospital in chaos and confusion. There were patients lying on the floor with anything from fractures and minor burns to life-threatening injuries and serious inhalation problems. I immediately took charge and organized a triage system with the nursing staff, working all that day and night. When I eventually arrived home exhausted the following morning, my guards were gone. Once again nursing saved me.

★★★

Just when life was becoming a little more bearable for us all, twenty-six-year-old Farah was arrested. The military police burst into the house and falsely accused him of deserting his unit several weeks earlier. As a lieutenant with two pips he faced a court martial and possible execution, which would leave my mother, pregnant sister and I broken and destitute.

The grounds for his arrest were so spurious it was laughable and related to a day when his entire convoy couldn't get through to a camp due to a cholera epidemic so they had no choice but to turn around and come back. We were in no doubt that he was really being arrested because of his relationship to me and to Mohamed. For his so-called 'crime' he was kept in solitary confinement for six months and I had to hire a lawyer to defend him. To make matters even worse, just as his court martial began my twenty-one-year-old sister was on the brink of delivering her first baby. That morning I left her in the hospital and ran to the court to try to find out what was happening. When I realized there was nothing I could see or do for my brother, I hurried back to my sister. In my absence Asha's life and that of her baby had been put in danger. An untrained midwife had mistakenly given her an intramuscular injection of oxytocin to boost her contractions – something that is never done during pregnancy as it can cause uterine rupture. Terrified that I might lose both my siblings – the one to medical and the other to military malpractice – I called her Sudanese doctor who immediately took her to the operating theatre and gave her anaesthesia to relax her stressed uterus and allow her to go into labour again. To my great relief, Asha eventually gave birth to a healthy baby boy, my nephew Mohamed. I was the one who delivered him.

There was more good news the following day – my honour student brother was acquitted of all charges and was waiting for me by the time I arrived home. It was a miraculous end to the most frightening few days of my life. The bad news was that, although he was a free man, Farah had been dismissed from the Army with no recompense, so both of us were out of work. My family was as poor as mud again, and I had no idea if I'd be allowed to do anything to save the situation. Secretly, I wondered if it was time to ask for my confiscated passport to be returned so that I could seek asylum in another country and pursue my career without oppression, but I also immediately knew that Siad Barre would never let me leave the country.

The event that changed things for the better was thanks to a vehicle. With all that had happened, I'd completely forgotten that before I left for London with Mohamed what seemed like years earlier, I had put down a deposit of 10,000 shillings on a brand new Toyota tipper truck that I planned to sub-contract out to create some income. The deposit was worth around $1,600, which I persuaded the dealer to return to me. Knowing that this money would be eaten up with our expenses, I wanted to make it work and earn us something, so I applied for a licence to run a dispensary and an ante- and post-natal consulting facility that I planned on calling the Mother and Child Health Clinic. I filled in all the applications and paid the fees only to receive a notification that the 'socialist' government had banned private clinics. I did, however, gain approval to dispense medicines, and in the Maka Mukarama district of Mogadishu I opened the Mother and Child Pharmacy, which quickly became known to all as the Edna Pharmacy.

I examined pregnant women in a room at the back of the premises and occasionally helped deliver their babies in their homes or referred them to hospital when necessary. Naturally, they'd also ask me to look at a child who was coughing or had a rash, dress a wound or give an injection, so my pharmacy became a mother and child clinic by default. Working there brought back so many memories of my days delivering babies at homes in south London and I drew on those lessons during these 'outlaw' days in Mogadishu. Six months after opening my pharmacy, which was by then thriving, two officials arrived to inform me of a new regulation that turned all private pharmacies into government co-operatives. My business and several others in the neighbour-hood were grouped into an International Pharmacy in the 'spirit of scientific socialism'. Overnight, I had six total strangers as business partners.

To this day, the district where I had operated my business is still known as 'Edna Pharmacy' as if it is a place name, in the same way that Hargeisa Group Hospital is still remembered by some as the Adan Ismail Hospital. These were things that Siad Barre could do nothing about.

In spite of my valuable work, the government still considered me a bourgeois dissident and continued to harass me. Every citizen of our country was obliged to attend political orienta-tion centres at least once a week to learn more about scientific socialism. Each community had its own centre, to which different groups would be summoned for special indoctrination sessions. After forced conscription was introduced for all male citizens from teenage years to middle age, they also received their initial training there. These buildings were plastered with huge posters of the world's greatest revolutionaries such as Karl Marx, Fidel Castro, Chairman Mao, Kim Il-sung, Che Guevara and Lenin, along with images of our 'great leader'. Some were lifelike oil paintings created by Communist lackeys in North Korea. These hung along aside the portraits of Siad Barre, which every office was obliged to have on its wall.

One of our indoctrination tasks was to prepare for the annual 21 October parade: an all-day event marking the date Barre bullied his way to power. In a huge parade ground on the edge of the city, known as Salaanta, which means salute, children called the 'flowers of the revolution' were trained for months by North Korean and East German officials to perform synchronized dance routines. On the day, they'd be marched out in their school uniforms to put on meticulously orchestrated displays of adoration for Barre while the women or 'mothers of the revolution' were required to sing along. Farmers would be marched in with their hoes and spades, and fishermen pulling a boat on wheels. Anthems would be sung, flags waved and flowers thrown, as a massive show of military might was rolled out showcasing Russian tanks and weaponry. Waves of planes flew overhead and endless columns of soldiers in military khaki with gold braid marched in perfect unison.

At one of my first special orientation sessions in a street that had been renamed October Road, I was surprised to find General Boots himself ready to address me and all the other pharmacy owners on the evils of capitalism. We were expected to sing our new national anthem, praising Barre as the saviour of our nation and wish him a long life. Seizing my moment, I moved to the front of our group and positioned myself right in front of him as I listened to his every hollow word. 'What you are doing is bad,' he lectured, wagging a finger at us. 'You are bleeding sick people for money. This is not in the spirit of our new nation.' Every so often he would suddenly cry, 'Long live the revolution!' at which point we were supposed to repeat the slogan and applaud. Whenever this happened, I would make eye contact with the man who'd left boot polish all over my carpets and furniture, the man who'd probably ordered the shooting of my dear Sanu, and who'd imprisoned my husband, and I very deliberately placed my hands behind my back.

Staring him out, making sure that he had noticed, my expression said, 'What can you do to me? You have taken all that I have. Do you want to be seen to punish a woman for not applauding you?' It was my way of protesting – my little piece of defiance. I couldn't tell from his stony expression if it bothered him or not, but it certainly made me feel better.

Another thing he couldn't stop me from doing around that time was entering the Mogadishu car rally, not long after I came out of house arrest in 1970. My Fiat 132 had recently been returned to me after I'd appealed to the authorities on the grounds that I was doing vital healthcare work. Not long afterwards, I heard an announcement on the radio inviting drivers to register for the rally around the streets of Mogadishu and my spirits soared. The regulations stipulated that each vehicle should have 'a driver and a female companion' – the assumption being that the driver would be male because hardly any women drove in Somalia. I immediately registered myself as 'E. Adan Ismail', the driver of my Fiat 132, with my brother's wife Layla Yusuf as my companion. On the morning of the rally I donned a shirt, trousers and a baseball cap to disguise my femininity, and drove to the starting line where I revved my car's engine like all the other competitors. The race began and off we went on a tortuous route that ran for at least ten kilometres through the back streets of the capital. The finishing line was in the football stadium where we had to complete different tasks in front of Siad Barre and his politburo, along with thousands of cheering Somalis.

In one of the events Layla, an air hostess who'd also learned to drive, had to jump out of our car and fill it with five litres of fuel against the clock, then feed me as many bananas and as much ice cream as she could in the allotted time. Anyone watching us from afar would have thought we were just a couple of skinny Somali men. Once we'd completed our tasks we had to race around the stadium and, once they took into account our rally time as well, we were ranked fifth out of fifty contestants, which delighted us as the first five winners were eligible for an award. Siad Barre himself came down onto the track to hand out the small trophies and, one by one, we winners had to climb the steps to the podium where he stood waiting. When it was my turn, I waited until I was standing right in front of him before pulling off my baseball cap. An official standing next to him saw his expression and immediately started stuttering, 'N–No, no, no, where is the driver?'

'I'm the driver,' I declared.

'No, no, that isn't allowed! You are disqualified! You cannot impersonate a man!'

'I did not impersonate a man,' I persisted. 'Your regulations only stipulated a driver. I am a driver who happens to be a woman, that's all.'

Exasperated, the official quickly conferred with his colleagues and spun back round to announce on the microphone, 'This driver is fined for impersonating a man. Points have been deducted and they are now in ninth place.' Turning back to me, he shouted, 'No prize!'

The cheers from the crowd when they saw who I was and realized what I'd done was the only prize I needed. Several of them even called out my name. Nodding to a seething Siad Barre I told him, 'You can keep your trophy', and left the podium with my hands raised in victory.

CHAPTER FOURTEEN

Mogadishu, Somalia, 1970

Frustrated at not hearing anything from Mohamed for over a year and convinced that he wasn't receiving my letters, I decided to try to send him a message some other way. I wanted to let him know that I was in Somalia, free to move about, and thinking of him.

Taking a male cousin along with me in case I was arrested, I drove my stalwart Fiat as close as I could to the high security compound in Afgoi where my husband was still imprisoned along with the rest of the pre-coup parliament and other prominent individuals. Rumours had been rife that they were going to be taken to court soon and then executed so I was extremely worried for him and for what our country had become.

Pulling up on a bridge over the Shebelle River just a few hundred metres from the fortress wall surrounding what had once been the country residence of the Italian Governor, I blocked a lane, stepped out of the car and unscrewed a tyre valve to let it run flat. Reaching into the vehicle, I pushed in a favourite cassette and turned the stereo up as loud as it would go to play our song, 'These Foolish Things' by Ella Fitzgerald. I then pulled off the volume knob and slipped it into my pocket.

Within minutes a policeman arrived who didn't recognize me and, although it was unusual to see a woman driving, his priority was to clear me from the highway. 'You have to move this car!' he told me as vehicles manoeuvered around me, hooting their horns.

'I can't. I have a puncture,' I told him, shrugging.

'Turn that music down!' he yelled, as the music blared out all around us.

'I've lost the knob. Look,' I said, pointing to the stereo.

'Do you have a jack?'

'What's that?' I asked, feigning ignorance.

By the time he'd found the jack and changed the wheel, my stereo had blasted out two or three songs long enough for Mohamed to hear them – or at least that's what I hoped. It was many years before I discovered that he had. Laughing, he knew that nobody else would have those songs on tape and that no one else would have been crazy enough to do what I did. Two or three weeks later I repeated the performance, driving there again to play exactly the same songs. I was lucky that a different policeman stopped me this time. As soon as Mohamed's fellow prisoners heard my stereo blasting Harry Belafonte's 'Island in the Sun', they ran to find him so that he could listen too. I would have done this every week but for the risk of being arrested too.

All I wanted was for my husband to be released so that we could pick up the pieces of our lives and start again. I had never stopped loving him and was fearful for both his safety and his welfare. Unfortunately for us, the government had no intention of releasing such a popular and influential figure so he remained behind concrete walls for four long years. It was only after the first three years that they finally allowed us to exchange letters but each was heavily censored and redacted. Anything that mentioned our situation or offered up any affection or complaint was blacked out, making little sense of what was written. What was left was like a shopping list of the things he wanted. I wasn't permitted to send Mohamed any food but he was allowed a few essentials, so I sent him a change of clothes and underwear and his pipe tobacco. He longed for books but I was only allowed to send him fiction, and no newspapers or magazines, so I bundled up anything I could lay my hands on, mostly novels in English such as Harold Robbins' *The Carpetbaggers* as well as some *Reader's Digest* condensed books. Mohamed told me later that even they often had pages torn out or blackened so as to frustrate him.

Trapped inside those high walls, he and his forty or so fellow prisoners were completely cut off from the world. They weren't beaten or tortured, but the mental torment was great. Family births, deaths and marriages happened without their knowledge. They filled their days with reading, prayer and meditation. They got into a routine and divided into their own groups but for all that time they had no idea what would come next or what was happening to their loved ones. Their only information came from authorities that manipulated the news to suit them.

The Siad Barre regime was not yet finished with me, either. My link to Mohamed kept me of interest to the regime and never far from suspicion. I would often find an unmarked car parked in our street with plain clothed policemen sitting inside, and I was still subject to random searches. The police seemed especially intrigued by the contents of my delivery bag kept in readiness for an emergency birth. They could recognize basic surgical instruments but were puzzled by the twisted white ligatures kept in alcohol to tie off umbilical cords. I told them they were worms to stop them from fishing them out with dirty fingers.

One day I returned home from work to find a man in civilian clothes standing outside my door. When he told me I was needed for an emergency I assumed he was a relative of one of my patients.

This was a regular occurrence for me, just as it had been for my father. It was only after we left the house that he informed me that he was an officer from the NSS and that I was under arrest. He ordered me to drive us both to the police station where they locked me in an empty office. After several hours alone, I was given some food served on a plate I recognized from home, so was comforted to know that Farah must have found out where I was being held. As night drew in the mosquitoes became unbearable so I banged on the door and demanded some bug spray. The police made me stand outside the room for ten minutes while it was sprayed before letting me back in. Then in the middle of the night I became desperate to use the toilet, so once again I called the guards. Smirking, they marched me to a cell full of male prisoners that had a single toilet without any door. The facilities were dirty and smelly but my bladder was bursting and this was my only option. As I prepared to relieve myself I glanced over my shoulder and saw that the men were watching. Rounding on them, I cried, 'Shame on you! Is this the kind of men you've become? I could be your wife or your sister or your mother. Show me the respect for privacy that you would want for them!' Some looked away but the rest sniggered until an older prisoner banged on the bars and commanded them to turn around with their backs to me. I was forever grateful to that man. As I was taken back to my 'cell' the police seemed frustrated that I hadn't been more embarrassed or humiliated and after that they let me use the commanding officer's personal toilet – with a door.

I had no idea why I'd been arrested or how long I'd be held this time. In the searing heat of the day they allowed me to sit outside in the shade of a mirimiri tree, whose twigs we Somalis use to brush our teeth. It wasn't until the third day that two plain-clothed police officers interrogated me along with three others who'd been arrested. Each of us had been kept in isolation, and none knew of the other.

The police's first question shocked me. 'How did you plan to kill Haile Selassie?'

My mouth dropped open and I laughed. 'Who? What are you talking about?'

'Haile Selassie, Emperor of Ethiopia.'

'I know who he is! He was a friend of my husband's. But why would I want to kill him?' The ridiculousness of their question took me by surprise, but their idiocy did not.

It soon became apparent that several leading African politicians were visiting Mogadishu in preparation for the Organization of African Unity Summit scheduled to convene there the following year. I discovered to my shock and amusement that I, along with several of Mohamed's colleagues from the parliamentary years, had been detained for supposedly plotting to assassinate Haile Selassie, who was to attend the summit. They clearly didn't want any of us 'anti-revolutionaries' to make contact with the visiting dignitaries. The whole idea was preposterous and undoubtedly came from some informer hoping to earn money from the authorities or at least remain in their good books.

'I may be many things but I am not in the assassination business,' I assured my interrogators. If the authorities had accused us of plotting to assassinate Siad Barre then that would have been far more plausible. After four days we were all released after signing documents promising that we wouldn't attempt to assassinate anyone. We were never charged with any crime, nor did we appear before any court. We were arrested merely to keep us from embarrassing the government in front of the VIP visitors.

Mohamed knew nothing of this, or of how difficult life was for my family and me. All that he'd been told by his captors was that I had opened a pharmacy and was making 'a lot of money'. In his isolation and paranoia, he became convinced that I must have sold everything we owned to fund it, not knowing that all our belongings had been taken by the government or looted by soldiers. Then I heard that he was communicating more openly with his first wife and asking her to send him things, which wounded me. The rock that broke the camel's back came when I wrote to ask him what he wanted me to do with his money I'd collected from the rent of his private house.

'Send it to my wife and children,' he wrote back.

'But I am your wife too!' I responded, expecting him to offer me a third or quarter and ask me to send the rest to his first family.

'This is my decision,' he replied. It was years before I learned that he'd been told that I was rolling in money while his children from his first marriage were starving. Not knowing this and failing to understand his reasoning, I did as he asked but wrote bitterly, 'Does this mean that I am no longer your wife?'

His answer broke my heart: 'Edna, you are as free as a bird.'

In a place where the prison guards deliberately doctored my letters to further fuel his suspicions, he became angrier and angrier in his responses to me. I was increasingly hurt by his unjustified accusations and frustrated by our inability to sit down and talk things through, as we should have. In such an impossible situation, there was no chance of reconciliation – there was only recrimination and sorrow. When he filed for divorce I couldn't contest it, as it is the prerogative of the husband, never the wife, to refuse or grant a divorce. I feel bad about it now and wish I had been more patient. The regime knew that we were stronger together and they deliberately split us up. To this day I regret playing into their hands.

★★★

Unexpectedly single again at thirty-five, I was still working as a midwife performing home deliveries and referring the most complicated cases to the Digfer Hospital where I'd done shifts as First Lady. It was there that I met a doctor called Federico Bartoli, who'd seen me work. Once we established that I didn't speak Italian and he didn't speak English, we found someone to interpret for us and he asked me if I was a doctor. When I explained that I was a midwife, he wanted to know where I had been trained. As soon as he learned that it was Britain, he invited me to work alongside him at the Italian-funded Medina police hospital, which served wealthy Somalis and expatriates as private patients.

The hospital had no maternity ward and no midwives, so delivering women there was a rather ad hoc affair and we had to improvise. It's best asset were the six Italian nuns who worked there without any nursing training but who were among the most dedicated and efficient staff I have ever worked with. Whenever a woman went into labour, the good doctor would summon me to his cramped office that had no running water or adjacent toilet, and move his desk aside in order for the mother to be wheeled in on a trolley. He and I would deliver the baby in that unsterile, unsuitable room, assisted by one of the nuns, and then mother and child would be moved to a ward. Once we were finished, a cleaner would come in to scrub the doctor's office and put it back the way it was.

Aside from the urgent need for a proper maternity ward with an appropriate delivery room, our biggest problem was the language barrier between us. Imagine my shock when – some months later – a Frenchwoman arrived at the hospital and greeted Dr Bartoli in her native tongue. To my surprise, he replied in perfect French.

When the visitor left, I turned to him incredulously, 'Dr Bartoli, *vous parlez français?*'

'*Bien sur, ma femme est française!*' I was as astounded as he was. It never occurred to him that someone from Somaliland who'd trained in Britain would speak French.

'For months, you made me speak in Italian,' I chastised. 'You didn't tell me that you spoke French!'

'You never asked me. You asked only if I spoke English, and I still don't.'

Now that we could converse freely we both agreed that the delivery arrangements at Medina were far from satisfactory, so Dr Bartoli persuaded the Italian government to build a new midwifery wing. When they agreed, he knew he needed some help. 'Why don't you design it for us, Edna?' he asked me. 'Make it just as you would like it.' He can't possibly have known that I had been dreaming of designing and building a hospital since I was a twelve-year-old girl, and had a blueprint ready and waiting in my head. Ever since I'd been cutting up bandages for my Dad I'd taken mental notes of when something worked or didn't, and I couldn't believe that I was finally going to be given the opportunity to put the best features into practice.

With the help of Dr Bartoli and an architect I immediately set about my task, sketching out my plans on a piece of paper from memory and experience. I summoned up the layouts of all the hospitals I'd been in that I'd liked, and those that I didn't. Being on the frontline, I knew firsthand what worked and what didn't and was thrilled to finally be able to put my experiences into practice. I insisted that the building be simple and efficient and I wanted the whole place to feel airy and light. It had to have a delivery area that could deal with two women at a time, a nearby sterilization area, and a lying-in ward. The Italians didn't follow all my instructions to the letter and it had several irritating features when it was completed, but it was a great improvement on Dr Bartoli's office. My favourite area was an east-facing verandah I designed between the kitchen and the main ward that had the perfect view of the sun peeping over the horizon early in the morning. It was also a lovely place to step out onto for a breather during night duty.

My design and diligence must have made an impression because once the prefab wing was complete the Italians then asked me to run the new unit. Then the Somali government reinstated my civil service appointment, on top of the salary I was earning from the hospital, so I was suddenly bringing in good money again – enough to comfortably support my family.

There were other big changes in my life too because, in 1973, four months after my marriage to Mohamed ended, I married again – this time to a civil servant named Ahmed Hussein Bulbul. I confess that I sank very low emotionally when my marriage ended and I remarried mostly out of spite. I knew it would hurt Mohamed and – at that point – I wanted to. He was still in prison and I still had feelings for him, but I couldn't help feel deeply wounded by his actions. I wanted him to think that I had moved on. Bulbul was a distant relative from the same clan, a friend of my brother's and a very good card player, playing rummy with my family on several occasions. An auditor in a government ministry, he'd been trained in Germany. Tall and handsome with salt and pepper hair, he was extremely eloquent in the Somali language. He was also articulate and intelligent and knew so much about poetry, history, and the old tribal ways. I had been on my own for many years by then so when he started to pay attention to me I was naturally flattered and welcomed human companionship. Even though Bulbul had already been married three times and had a child by each of them, when he told me one day, 'I love you and I'd like to marry you,' I heard myself say, 'Okay.'

With hindsight, our marriage was probably doomed from the start. Somali marriages typically include three stages. First, there is the formal request for the hand of the woman from her male relatives. Then there is the official betrothal or *meher*, registered in the presence of the sheikh, where the dowry is agreed. Finally, there is the marriage itself. The first two stages don't usually require the presence of the bride, just her male relatives – my brother and uncles. However, halfway through the *meher* I received a call from Dr Bartoli asking for my help with an emergency C-section. Without hesitating, I left the celebration and rushed to the hospital, scrubbed up, put on my gown, and joined the surgical team. In the middle of the procedure, I looked through the glass of the operating room and saw my brother, uncles and the sheikh tapping on the glass partition to get my attention.

A medical assistant went to speak with them at my request and returned with the message: 'Your family and the sheikh need your consent to the marriage with Bulbul.' As I was in the middle of assisting a new life into this world, I sent the assistant back with the message, 'Yes.'

He quickly returned. 'The sheikh insists he has to hear it from your own mouth.' Exasperated, I went over to the glass partition, had the assistant open the door for me and abruptly told him, 'Yes, yes', before waving them all away with bloodstained gloves. From that day on I was accused of having no respect for my marriage responsibilities by both my relatives and Bulbul's. In spite of my shortcomings, though, I was still the daughter of Adan Doctor and the fact that Bulbul was from my clan sent a message to them all that I was still considered valuable as a wife. From my perspective, marrying Bulbul meant that I could move with my

mother and sister into his larger government house and rent out
Mum's property for extra income. My brother moved next door
with his wife, so we were all together again.

Not long after my second marriage, I heard that Mohamed
had been released. I was relieved and happy for him, and a bit
sad too. Rather poignantly, my first sight of Mohamed after his
imprisonment was in a restaurant about a year after my marriage
to Bulbul. Mohamed was about to move to India, where the
authorities sent him as Somali Ambassador for two years, chiefly
to keep him out of the way. I didn't even know he was in the
same room until he walked over to our table to say hello. Placing
a hand on Bulbul's shoulder, he said, 'You take care of this girl.
I should have but I didn't, so make sure you do.' Nothing more
was said and it would be many years before Mohamed and I would
finally make our peace, but I was touched by his words, which
I interpreted as his apology to me.

Working at Medina was rewarding but also extremely frustrating
at times, such as the Superglue incident when I'd had to threaten
the director to ensure he provided my patients with the necessary
oxygen. That little girl survived, by the way, and I still have a piece
of crochet that she made for me in school. Her mother named
her Culus, which means 'heavyweight'. Time and again, though,
experiences like hers not only reminded me of the importance of
my work and how rewarding it is to save a life, but made me wish
I could build my own hospital and run it just the way I wanted to,
without the interference of politics, money or negative influences.

The midwifery ward where we had managed to save Culus's life
soon became the place that all the leading politicians and Italian
businessmen sent their wives and daughters rather than sending
them back to Rome to have their babies. I even delivered two of
President Siad Barre's daughters and both his wives were treated

there, whose medication I personally administered for fear that someone might poison them and I'd be shot for it. One of the saddest episodes from my time at Medina involved the first wife of Lieutenant-General Mohamed Ali Samatar, the Vice President and part of Barre's inner circle. A lovely woman from the old town of Barawe, she was due to deliver her tenth child but because she had had a history of heavy bleeding I advised her in a pre-natal visit to come in to the hospital as soon as she felt her first contractions. Strangely, I never saw her again.

Two weeks later, a soldier brought in a baby wrapped in a bloodstained blanket and told me it was Ali Samatar's daughter. One of the nuns helped me clean the infant as I tried to find out from the soldier where the mother was. Then Ali Samatar himself arrived to see how his newborn was doing. When I asked about his wife, he began to cry uncontrollably. 'She died,' he sobbed. I couldn't help but be moved by his pain. When his tears had dried, he asked me what he should do with the baby. I advised him to find someone he trusted, and I offered to train her to look after the baby. He returned to the hospital a few days later with his sister, and we prepared her to become the baby's foster mother.

It was some time before I discovered the details of what had happened. A midwife who was a relative of Siad Barre, and someone I had previously sacked from Medina for incompetence, had set herself up in private practice. It was she who had recommended to Samatar that his wife could be delivered at home, ignoring the fact that her patient was high risk with a history of excessive bleeding. As expected, the woman haemorrhaged after delivery and died before the Russian doctors summoned by Ali Samatar could get there. The poor woman must have lost a pint of blood per minute post-partum. Clearly the midwife was unprepared to deal with the complications.

Following Somali custom, Ali Samatar was given his deceased wife's sister to marry, and I would later deliver both her babies before I ended my time at Medina. Ali Samatar would go on to become Siad Barre's Defense Minister and finally Prime Minister. Under his watch in the 1980s, more than a quarter of a million of our people in Somaliland suffered heinous human rights violations: displacement, torture, civilian bombardment and mass executions. I owe it to those victims to acknowledge that Ali Samatar was a war criminal. The husband who'd wept openly for his beloved wife and sought care for his baby girl showed no mercy to the citizens of my country. Our paths would cross again later and Samatar did not forget my neutrality when it came to caring for the sick and needy, regardless of who they were, or who they were married to. As we say, God's rain falls equally on the just and the unjust.

***

Even though I was never the kind of conventional wife who would cook or clean or roll up Bulbul's socks, we were happy for our first year of marriage and it felt to be a good match. Like any Somali man, he'd occasionally complain that I didn't know where his clothes were or was wastefully hiring servants to do the housework I should have been doing but, to begin with at least, he handled my career better than Mohamed had.

What he did find difficult was the other, unexpected conse-quences of being married to me. Having never been monitored or arrested he suddenly found himself under constant police scrutiny. Then he was imprisoned, with me, for the first time in his life, which shocked him to the core. It happened shortly before my 38th birthday in September 1975. I had just returned from Rome and another inconclusive round of fertility tests, and Bulbul and I were taking a short holiday to Baligubadle, our clan village seventy kilometres south of Hargeisa, where his relatives were planning to slaughter a sheep in our honour. About eight kilometres from our destination, two police cars stopped our vehicle, told us to get out, and searched it from top to bottom. Without any explanation, they arrested us all and made us turn back to Hargeisa.

Bulbul and I were held in custody on the screened-in verandah of the police station for two days (while male prisoners leered at me from inside), and then taken somewhere else for a night before being locked into what felt like an airless container for six days. That's where I spent my birthday. Pacing our 'cell', Bulbul became convinced that our imprisonment was my fault and spent the entire week asking me, 'What did you say this time? What did you do?' On the seventh day, three plain-clothes police officers interrogated us separately about our 'plot' to escape from Somalia, which was laughable when I'd only just returned from Italy. Eventually, without any evidence and in the face of our persistent denials, they let us go.

The final straw for Bulbul and me came in January 1976, not long after our release. I was summoned to what I was told was an important meeting with the Minister of Health, who abruptly informed me that I was to be sent for mandatory military service at Halane. The camp had been turned into a boot camp and political orientation centre where discipline and revolutionary zeal was instilled in government officials, teachers and civil servants.

In preparation for my departure, I was escorted to the orienta-tion room at the Ministry and found it full of military person-nel and new inductees who, like me, had been unexpectedly conscripted. I heard them respond to those who were protesting that even pregnant women or people with one kidney still owed service to their country. I knew then that, as a fit thirty-eight-year old, there was no getting out of it. An officer handed out lists of regulations: men should cut their hair short and bring a change of athletic clothes. Women should cover their hair and wear tracksuits. Only one suitcase per person would be allowed, and no more than one hundred shillings or $13 in cash.

When I got home and told Bulbul that I was being sent to Halane, he couldn't believe it, and became convinced that I'd volunteered to get away from him. In a way, he was right. I probably could have refused to go on the grounds that my work was essential, but I would have had to beg and that wasn't my style. I had another reason for not refusing: I was determined to show the 'big boys' that I was no 'softie' and couldn't be intimidated, just as I had shown the little boys in the neighbourhood back when I was a kid.

As soon as I arrived at the camp twenty-four hours later, I took a top bunk near a window. We were ordered to pick out our uniforms in an old airplane hangar filled with mountains of used Soviet military uniforms, unwashed khaki shirts and trousers with holes. I wear size 37 shoes but had to settle for size 40, the smallest they had. I figured that I could wear layers of socks that would also pad my feet for all the marching I was expecting to do. I didn't realize double socks also meant double heat when the outside temperature was already in the 30s. I later learned to stuff cotton wool into my boots to fill the empty space beyond my toes. Our first job was to wash the stink of sweat and mould out of our uniforms, polish our shoes and the brass buttons of our uniforms, tasks I did with resolve to demonstrate that I was well accustomed to scrubbing and polishing and they weren't teaching me anything new.

There were just over two hundred in our platoon, and from the start we competed with each other in everything from physical

stamina to our revolutionary commitment. A typical day started
at 04:00 hours when we were awoken by shrill whistles. We ran
and did gymnastics until 06:00, took showers, then put on our
uniforms for breakfast before an hour of marching drill. There
were also daily indoctrination sessions in which we were given
lectures on the history and glories of scientific socialism and
communism compared with the evils of capitalism. Our work
details involved projects reclaiming land from sand dunes, setting
up and dismantling tents at speed, painting old warehouses and
clearing vast rubbish dumps. With all the daily exercise, including
running and stretching, Halane was fantastic physical training.
I have never been in better shape, even though I gained three
kilos from eating so heartily at a time when most of my comrades
lost weight. For them, Halane was four months of hell but I never
complained, as this was my way of resisting.

We endured all this for forty days until we were allowed to
leave the camp for the first time. My next work detail was being
assigned to a committee building dormitories for soldiers. We
had to raise funds from patriotic citizens and businessmen and
then collect the construction materials from local suppliers. I used
my car, which I'd been allowed to keep, and they allocated me
five litres of fuel per trip to run around town and find what we
needed. Another of my responsibilities was to deliver the babies
of officers' wives, including that of the general in command. One
night at 21:00 hours while standing to attention in full khaki
uniform for the final roll call, the commander summoned me out
of line. The Halane camp doctor needed to speak to me. I had
previously helped deliver his sister's babies by C-section, and he
told me she was now at the Medina undergoing another long and
difficult labour. 'The doctor there says she can have this child
naturally, but you told her that any further births would have

to be delivered surgically or it would be too dangerous for her and the baby. Please can you go and see her?' He added that the baby was very big and when he told me the name of the doctor I genuinely feared for her as – although he was from an important clan he was medically incompetent – I wouldn't have allowed him to deliver my donkey. Phoning ahead, I told the nuns to prepare the theatre and call the anaesthetist, as the patient would need a Caesarian. Still in my army uniform and boots, I got into the doctor's car and had him drive me to the hospital.

As soon as I examined his sister I knew that she would rupture unless she had immediate surgery and I told the sister to summon the doctor urgently. When he arrived he instructed me to stimulate her contractions, which I knew was a dangerous mistake. 'Do you really want me to do that?' I asked. 'You know that she previously had a C-section?' He insisted so I made him write down his instructions so that I wouldn't be blamed if something went wrong. Unfazed, he did as I asked and said he'd check that the theatre was ready. I started a slow drip that immediately stimulated strong contractions, so I stopped it and went to find him. That's when I discovered that he had left the hospital. His car was gone and the guards told me he had driven through the gates some time ago. There was no reply at his house either so there I was, stranded in the middle of the night, without a doctor capable of performing this emergency surgery. I had no choice but to call for the inexperienced duty doctor to deliver the baby via forceps. By the time we got it out, the child was dead and we had to cut the woman extensively to extract its body. I was so angry at this senseless loss of life that I wrote up my report of everything that had happened, attaching the incompetent doctor's written orders. At the end of my report I proclaimed that I wouldn't set foot in Medina hospital again until the doctor involved had been removed from medical service. He never was and so I never did.

When Bulbul heard through the grapevine that I had been driven from Halane in the middle of the night by a male doctor, he immediately assumed I was having an affair. He objected to what he saw as my 'unwifely behaviour' and complained once more that I always put my patients first. He used to tell people, 'I'm Edna's secretary, launderer, blood bank and coffee maker but she has no time to be my wife.' In fairness, he had a point.

Just like my father I was always on call for hospital emergencies. As they had done with my father when I was a little girl, people would come to our house at all times of the day or night to summon me or enquire after their relatives. One night the hospital sent an ambulance to collect me at the Cinema Centrale where Bulbul and I had gone for a rare night off. The manager stopped the film to find me, which greatly embarrassed my husband. When I eventually arrived home much later that night, he muttered angrily, 'You shouldn't have told the hospital where you were.'

Little did he know how deeply Dad's selflessness was ingrained in me when it came to those in need, or how far I was prepared to go in campaigning for better healthcare for everyone in my country. Like my father, who was the hardest act to follow, I was married to the hospital and no one else could ever match up to it.

★★★

The authorities must have been impressed that I didn't try to wriggle out of Halane and did all that was expected without complaint, because they almost immediately gave me a senior civil servant position. That is how schizophrenic the regime was. Or perhaps they simply knew my weakness was healthcare and decided to use it to their advantage.

Either way, no sooner had I returned from boot camp than

I was summoned by the Minister of Health and offered the post of Director of Human Resources Development for Health in his ministry. It was the first time a woman had been put in charge of what was a new ministerial department. I was responsible for the professional training and my priorities were to monitor, evaluate and, where necessary, upgrade the curriculum in each programme. I also had to assess the performance of nurses, midwives, laboratory technicians, pharmacists, sanitarians, and public health professionals working in government facilities and arrange for their in-service training.

My office became like a market place as I was swamped with visitors, meetings, seminars, complaints and paperwork. As if we didn't have enough to do, every Monday my colleagues and I had to undergo political orientation sessions on scientific socialism run by the *Guudida Shaqaalaha,* the workers' committee. In a large conference hall we were instructed to enthusiastically sing revolutionary songs praising Comrade Siad Barre, as well as learning lists of regulations to abide by. One of these regulations stated that because the fighting in the Ogaden region was heating up as the regime prepared to launch a war against Ethiopia, all of us department directors were to organize a rota so that one of us remained on duty every night to respond to any emergencies and deal with casualties from the front. Partly because my marriage was disintegrating, but mainly because I wanted to catch up with my work, I was happy to take part. That one evening each week was my time to concentrate, write, think and be creative. The others, all men, treated their evening shifts as a boys' night out, bringing in khat to chew with the security guards downstairs as they argued about politics, listened to music and generally had a good time. Khat is a plant in the bittersweet family and has become the scourge of our country. Once chewed it releases a stimulant that induces feelings of euphoria in the same way as amphetamines. All across East Africa people are addicted and, in my opinion, nobody who is chewing khat can be doing their job to the best of their ability.

At one of the Monday orientation sessions, a member of the workers' committee publicly denounced me. 'I think you should know,' he declared, 'that a certain director who thinks of herself as above the others, locks herself in her air-conditioned office whenever she's on evening duty and refuses to associate with the staff.' Furious, I jumped to my feet and protested that I worked longer hours than anyone else and was merely doing my job – waiting by the telephone ready to organize casualties at a moment's notice. For good measure, I added, 'As you've brought up the air-conditioning when I don't even have a fan in my office, I would now like it to be installed.'

The following week I did as I always did and worked my tail off alone in my office well beyond midnight, only to be told at the next orientation session that I was not following the ethos of Barre's Revolutionary Socialist Party. At the end of the month I was fined three days' salary – for doing the right thing. My response was to refuse to turn up for any of my appointed shifts, but to be there any other night of the week. Nobody dared do a thing about my private rebellion and no one mentioned it again or fined me for my open disobedience.

As Director of Health Training I made several trips to the north to inspect and evaluate the Ministry's training programme in Somaliland, give talks to health personnel, and hold final exams for student nurses. What I discovered there in 1977 horrified me. The nine-month Ogaden War started by Barre that summer was already proving to be a disaster chiefly because the Soviets had changed their mind about him, abandoned Somalia, and were reinforcing their other allies including Ethiopia. Against such opposition, a third of the Somali National Army invasion force was killed and half of our Air Force destroyed.

From the moment I arrived in Hargeisa, I was inundated with requests for help. The casualties from the front had been evacuated to empty warehouses converted into makeshift hospitals in the Ganat area in the hills overlooking the city. Then the most seriously injured were transported to Hargeisa General Hospital where the nursing staff reported that they were dying in their hundreds. Several soldiers lost limbs simply because tourniquets had been mistakenly left applied for days. I went to see the situation in Ganat for myself and was appalled by what I found. Besides motivating my nurses and midwives to be more proactive, I also offered to train the soldiers in First Aid so that when one of them was injured, they knew what measures to take to avoid complication and possible amputations of limbs that could have been healed and saved. I had a vested interest as my brother Farah had been re-conscripted into the military and was fighting at the front somewhere near the Kenyan border.

I was sent to see Siad Barre's deputy, Ali Samatar, by then Minister of Defence and chief commanding officer of the army. The man whose wife had died at home because of an inept midwife agreed that his troops urgently needed to acquire some medical skills, suspecting rightly that the conflict would develop into a full-scale war. With his blessing, I spent the next two weeks training forty soldiers in first aid to treat injuries in the field. I was assisted in my quest by an unexpected ally – Hassan Kayd, my childhood friend and the soldier whose life I'd saved after the abortive military coup. It was good to see him. The last time we'd met was when he'd advised us on security at our home in the Lido what seemed like a hundred years earlier. Now he was back in uniform as the colonel in charge whose cooperation I needed. I think Hassan always felt indebted to me for having saved his skin and he made sure I had everything I required including daily military transportation to the military camp at Dararweyne, in the middle of nowhere, some forty kilometres out of town.

Following a heavy battle between rival forces at the border regions of Jigjiga, Karamara, and almost as far as Harar, the army commander asked me to accompany a junior doctor and evacuate the most seriously injured from the front. I agreed readily, eager to see for myself the conditions there. We left at night and were driven there in a military lorry with its headlights off to avoid becoming another target for the Ethiopian air force. A mechanic who accompanied us sat up front, using his torch to help navigate the rutted dirt tracks and treacherous potholes. As we approached Jigjiga we could hear the sounds of guns and heavy artillery that told us how close we were to the fighting. An armed escort took us into the military compound.

The sight that greeted me in the warehouses was one of the most horrendous I have ever seen. I could smell the two hundred or so patients long before I could see them. They lay on the floor of the vast building in their own filth, their wounds festering without anyone to care for them and hardly any medical supplies. If I could, I'd have evacuated them all but the truck only had room for fifty of the most critical patients and then only the ones I decide could survive the arduous trip. Deciding who to leave behind was one of the hardest decisions I've ever had to make. I will never forget the expressions on the faces of those I chose not to take.

Waiting until nightfall, we drove back along roads so bumpy that the soldiers frequently cried out in-pain. It was excruciating for them without any sedatives or painkillers. The stink of their gangrenous wounds filled our vehicle. Halfway through our journey, the lorry lurched violently to one side when a tyre burst on a rock. As our mechanic jumped out and tried to repair it by flashlight, we could see the glowing eyes of hyenas approaching in the dark, lured by the smell of human flesh, which they had been feeding on freely from the battlefields. That was without a doubt the scariest moment of my life.

'What have I done?' I asked myself, close to panicking. 'I've saved these patients from that terrible compound only to see them torn apart by hungry hyenas!' The soldiers were far too sick and weak to protect us or themselves and we had just one weapon with us, which I only then learned was loaded with a single bullet. Defenceless, we banged on the sides of the truck with rocks and shouted at the beasts each time they drew closer. Allah be praised, the driver and the mechanic somehow changed the wheel and we set off again to safety.

CHAPTER FIFTEEN

Mogadishu, Somalia, 1977

I returned to Mogadishu and my failing marriage little know-ing that my efforts to save lives on the frontline were only the prelude to what would become the toughest and most challenging campaign of my life – the battle to end female circumcision.

My opportunity to act had first come in 1976 when the Ministry sent me to attend a WHO congress on obstetrics and gynaecol-ogy in Khartoum, Sudan, with two male gynaecologists. There were at least four hundred participants at the event, including doctors, religious leaders and midwives, but what I remember most were the numbers of traditional clan elders in turbans, robes and beards alongside female activists. Many issues were on the agenda relating to obstetrics and gynaecology, including diseases of the reproductive organs, childbirth complications and sexually transmitted diseases. Towards the end of the congress, a Sudanese doctor named Dr Taha Ahmed Baasher, then serving as WHO's Regional Adviser on Mental Health, stood up and gave a presentation. I couldn't have been more stunned if someone had thrown a bucket of camel milk over me. There I was, sitting in a packed auditorium alongside two Somali men, listening to a learned colleague talking openly about about the medical and psychological complications of female circumcision – a subject we never, ever discussed in public back home and certainly never between men and women. To compound my shock, Dr Baasher had an accompanying slideshow in which he calmly presented close-up images of the female anatomy on a huge screen, illustrating the various forms of circumcision practised across Africa.

Once I got over the initial shock, I realized that he was describing exactly what I had gone through and had been observing daily in my maternity wards. 'My God,' I thought, 'I had no idea this was so widespread.' My heart was beating hard against my ribcage as my brain tried to take in all that I was hearing. I had no idea what I was going to do with this information or how I might ever be able to present it to a Somali audience but my head was spinning with possibilities. When I flew back to Mogadishu with my colleagues, none of us said a word about what we'd just heard and seen. We sat together on the plane, avoiding the subject and too embarrassed to speak about it, making small talk instead.

Some weeks after my return the Minister of Health called me into his office to tell me that the following week the government was organizing a congress of women to launch a new organization, the Somali Women's Democratic Organisation. Various ministries had been invited to present initiatives targeting women's contribution to the development of Somalia and to scientific socialism. 'As the only female director in the Ministry of Health, you have the pleasure and responsibility to talk to your women,' he told me with a smile.

'Okay, Comrade Minister, what would you like me to talk about?'

Knowing that we'd have a captive audience, he replied, 'Oh, the usual things, Edna – immunizations, measles, whooping cough – whatever you'd like.'

Until that moment, I had never imagined broaching the subject of female circumcision with this man, or any man, but I heard myself suddenly blurt, 'Well, Mr Minister, if it is really up to me then I will talk about female circumcision.' That was the first time those words had ever left my mouth.

The Minister literally jumped back in his seat and said, 'Edna! What has come over you? You can't talk about something like that!' I knew him very well; I'd delivered three of his kids and we had mutual respect for one another. Still, I could see his dismay. 'Are you forgetting who you are?' he added, his expression one of horror. 'You are the daughter of Adan Ismail, you cannot speak about this in public. Please, don't even consider it!'

Shaking my head, I told him, 'Mr Minister, it is *because* I am the daughter of Adan Ismail that I must speak about it. If I don't, then who will?'

He did everything he could to talk me out of it. When begging didn't work he tried to scare me. 'They'll… they'll throw shoes at you,' he stuttered. 'They'll spit at you. The women will never listen to you. Talk about something else, Edna, I beg you. How about breastfeeding, or polio, or any of the other subjects you like to talk about?'

'No, Comrade,' I replied, my mind made up. 'I've talked about those things quite enough. This time I am going to talk about female circumcision.' I knew in my heart from that moment on there was no going back. This was the right time. The subject wasn't going to be locked in the closet again. It needed to be brought out into the open and I had to be the one to do it, even if – secretly – I wasn't sure if I'd have the courage and competence to go through with it convincingly.

Since my boss couldn't persuade me to change my mind, he settled for a compromise. Sighing, he said, 'Why don't you bring me an outline of what you want to talk about, and I'll think about it.'

'You'll have it in the morning,' I replied, far more confidently than I felt.

I returned to my office and thought back to what Dr Baasher had said in Khartoum about the health risks of female circumcision. I knew that I would be talking to a non-medical Somali audience, who would never have heard the subject discussed publicly before. I needed some advice. When I was married to Mohamed I'd discuss everything with him, so when I went home for lunch, I raised the subject with Bulbul.

My husband's mouth fell open. 'What are you saying?' he cried. 'You can't talk about that!'

'I can and I must,' I replied. 'But first I want your help. I need you to tell me what a man really feels about this.' To my surprise, Bulbul became an ally. It was he who suggested I talk with somebody knowledgeable about the religious aspect of circumcision and he called Yaxye Sheikh Ibrahim, a friend of his, who came to our house. For the third time that day, I found myself talking to a man about this taboo subject. Fortunately, the friend wasn't shocked to learn of my feelings and confirmed that the Qur'an does not require the practice. For Muslim boys circumcision is obligatory, but there are no Qur'anic directives for girls. Helpfully, he gave me a quotation from our Prophet Muhammad, peace be upon him. When *Umm Atiya*, a woman who performed circumcisions on Arab women, asked the Prophet what Muslims should do, he replied, 'Touch, but do not cut.' It seemed to be an explicit instruction not to circumcise women, although many use this to claim that it is recommended or even obligatory.

With this information in my armoury, I finished the draft of my presentation and handed it to the Minister the following morning. He was on his way out of the office to meet with the President, but took my document and promised to get back to me. When he returned a couple of hours later, he said, 'You want to talk about this? Go ahead.' His dramatic change of heart made me suspicious, especially after he'd spent so long trying to discourage me. There had to be a catch. Then I realized what it was. Siad Barre and I were sworn enemies; he saw me as a dissident anti-revolutionary who stood against everything he represented. He frequently ordered that my house be searched and sent police to detain me. But he also knew that I was popular with the public and there would be outrage if anything serious happened to me. All he could do was give me a little pinch now and then, like putting me in jail for a few days to demonstrate his annoyance or to remind me of his power. When the Minister told Barre of my intentions to talk publicly about circumcision, the President must have seen it as a gift from God. 'Let her talk about un-talkable things,' he told him. 'She will be shamed in the eyes of the people. Edna Adan Ismail will be cutting her own throat.'

I thanked the Minister for bringing me the President's approval and then dropped my next bombshell. 'And, of course, you must be there when I make my speech.' He almost fell over at the suggestion.

'No, no, no!' he objected. 'We didn't agree to that. If you want to do this then you have my permission, but you will be the only one who talks about – *that*.' He couldn't even bring himself to use the words.

I shook my head. 'No, Mr Minister. I am going to the conference as a director of the Ministry. I'll be speaking about what you have authorized me to speak about. You must be there in your capacity as a minister.'

'But I can't, Edna!' he pleaded. 'I'm a man! I can't be in the room when you talk about that part of the body!'

I tutted. 'Mr Minister, you are the Minister of Health – even for

that part of the body.' When he continued to protest I threatened
to talk about measles or polio or immunizations instead, which
I knew was not what the President would now want to hear. We
argued the point for several minutes until he finally conceded,
'Alright, Edna, I'll come. I will open the seminar, I'll introduce
you and then I'll walk out.' I wasn't letting him off that lightly
and told him that as soon as he walked out, I would change the
subject. In the end, he had no choice but to agree to my plan.

★★★

The conference was held at the police academy. When we arrived
we found the building surrounded by officers armed with shields
and sticks. This wasn't the norm for every government meeting
and I was told that the riot police had been mobilized because
the authorities believed people would rebel when I started to
speak. After sitting through the opening ceremonies with great
trepidation, I was introduced by the Minister. I walked up to
the podium, took a deep breath and began: 'Women, I will be
talking to you today about a subject of the greatest importance.
You are accustomed to hearing from me about many health issues.
Remember when I told you about immunizations but when it
came time to do them you hid your children under your beds?
Now that everyone knows the importance of protecting children
against diseases, mothers stand in long lines to get their children
immunized, so we have come a long way. Do you remember
when you'd go through pregnancies without ever being examined
and there would be complications? Now many women come for
check-ups throughout their pregnancies. I am so grateful that you
have taken all of our advice.

'Today, I am going to talk to you about another problem and

I not only need your help, I need you to take this advice just as
you have in the past. The subject that I'm going to talk about is
not going to be comfortable, but it is one that affects our women,
it affects me and you, it affects the births of our children, it affects
the wellbeing of our daughters. It causes pain, it causes bleeding...'
As I built up the suspense, the audience must have been wondering
what new disease I was going to discuss. I could almost sense their
minds trying to figure it out. It was time to put them out of their
misery. 'The subject that I have been describing, the thing which
causes all of these problems for you and me... is the circumcision
of our girls.' A shock wave rippled around the conference hall
and there were several audible gasps. Almost every woman in the
auditorium lowered her head and tugged on her head covering.

'You are doing exactly what I thought you'd do!' I told them.
'You are hiding. You are ashamed of hearing me talk about this.
Believe me, I, too, am ashamed but I have no option. I need to
talk – we need to talk about this as responsible adults who care
for our children. You need to listen to me, and you need to
understand. I'm not talking about something that you do not
know. I know that you have gone through this, as I have gone
through it. Every single one of us has experienced this and it is
time to talk about it.'

I barely took a breath as I kept the momentum going and spoke
of the bleeding, the difficulties with urination, the complications
during childbirth and about all the infections I had come across.
'There must be women out there – in this very audience – who are
older than I am and who have much more experience than I have
on this subject. And if there are, I want them to talk to us, too.'
One by one, the heads came up. They were curious. They were
listening. I could see a few women nodding. They were attentive
and absorbed. The Minister, who'd been squirming in his seat,

saw this too and suddenly appeared very interested, ready to take credit for introducing the subject that had everyone buzzing.

I paused before pleading, 'If there is anyone out there with something to say, then please, let us hear from you.' After a slight hesitation, a little old woman sitting at the back of the auditorium put up her hand. She got up from her seat and started to walk slowly towards the stage. 'Yes, yes, come to the podium,' I encouraged. 'Come closer to the microphone.'

Once at the front, she began to speak. 'I am an old woman; I don't know how old I am. But I am very old. To show you how old I am, I am going to let you see my white hair, which nobody has seen except for my husband.' She lifted her headdress to reveal hair the colour of cotton. 'This is how old I am. And all the time that this white hair was growing on my head, I wanted to talk about this.' Turning to me, she added, 'What you are talking about has been done to me. I bled and I suffered and I became infected.' Without pausing she talked about all the medical problems she'd dealt with after her cutting and then she said, 'My daughter went through it also. She, too, experienced these things. And only recently, my granddaughter has lived through this and suffered also. I am grateful that I have been spared from the grave to see this day and to talk about this terrible practice.'

That old woman really saved the day. Everybody applauded and some even gave her a standing ovation. Their response encouraged another woman to put her hand up and cry, 'I also have a problem!' Others followed. Before calling for a short recess, I decided to shock them with the revelation that female circumcision wasn't universal. 'Muslims in the Sudan do not practise it, nor do women in Saudi Arabia,' I told them as they stared at me in surprise. I quoted the verse from the Qur'an that said, 'Don't cut', and asked why we Somalis were among the few Muslim countries that went against the teachings of Islam. I then asked them to group together according to their regions and select one spokesperson from each. 'When we come back from our break, we will hear from all sixteen regions. Tell us what you think about circumcision. Do we fight it and continue to talk about it or do we leave it and stay silent about it? We want you to tell us what you want.' During the tea break women accosted me from all sides – not rebelling or angry as the authorities may have hoped, but firing questions at me and congratulating me on what I had done. When we reconvened, they had so much to say that I had to limit them to five minutes each. That day in March 1976 truly marked the beginning of our struggle against female circumcision. We launched the Somali Women's Democratic Organization and formed a national committee to address women's issues.

Not that talking about female circumcision elsewhere was as easy as at that conference. Many, many people criticized us and claimed that our ideas were the result of pernicious Western influences. We insisted that the campaign wasn't a Western plot and was initiated by us. 'Women in the West do not undergo circumcision,' I protested. 'We Africans are the ones who feel the pain and suffer the haemorrhages, the infections and the problems. This is our struggle and it is for us to find our own solution to it.'

In the forty plus years since I first broached the subject, I have been tirelessly campaigning against female circumcision. I've represented Somalia and later Somaliland at so many conferences on the subject that I have lost count. I went back to Khartoum in 1979, and then I teamed up with Sudanese colleagues for presentations in Senegal and Egypt under the auspices of the World Health Organization. I have spoken in the US and in Geneva, all over the Netherlands including Amsterdam and The Hague, in Britain, across Scandinavia and Germany. I became the chief adviser on female circumcision for the WHO's regional office in the Mediterranean region, which is where we first coined the term Female Genital Mutilation or FGM to replace the more benign female circumcision. I was privileged to participate in the Fourth World Conference on Women in Beijing in 1995. America's First Lady Hillary Clinton was in attendance as were the First Ladies of Ghana and Egypt, the Queen of Jordan, and the activist and actress Jane Fonda, among others. After the opening speeches, I was the first person to raise my hand and ask, 'And what is the world going to do about female genital mutilation? Women will never go forward while this practice goes on.' After I'd finished speaking, Jane Fonda came down from the stage and shook my hand.

The fight against female circumcision has come a long way but it is far from over. It will certainly take longer than the lifetime of one stubborn midwife to achieve its ultimate goal. The percentage of women affected is still far too high but, according to the latest figures we obtained from the study we made at the Edna Adan Teaching Hospital, a quarter of our female population has at least been spared (this study in its entirety can be accessed on the hospital website: www. ednahospital.org).

One of the tactics we are using now is to engage and educate men about FGM. It has always been considered a women's issue only, but it is time to make it everybody's problem from the grandfather to the father to the religious leader. We need to show them pictures of female circumcision to prove to them how radically different it is to male circumcision, as many of them naively assume. My father was appalled by what had been done to me because he'd seen the results of FGM as a doctor. He knew of the pain and the possible complications I faced. If we make other men aware of this and enlist them to courageously join the battle then I feel sure that we will start to reduce the numbers.

One new problem is that the practice is spreading around the world as Somalis and other women from our continent have emigrated or been forced to flee. In Britain and the US midwives like me are coming across all the associated complications with the women they are delivering, and having to deal with them for the first time. They also face legal battles if doctors need to operate as it can be considered a 'violation' of a woman's virginity. When Theresa May was the UK's Home Secretary I met with her and begged her to make FGM illegal in Britain so as to stop the practice from spreading. In 2012, the United Nations adopted a worldwide ban, calling FGM 'an irreparable and irreversible abuse' of human rights. They also set up an International Day of Zero Tolerance for FGM, and in 2018 Africa's first female president, Liberia's Ellen Johnson Sirleaf, formally outlawed FGM in her country on her final day in office.

Throughout my campaign, I have chosen my words carefully and deliberately tried to limit myself to focusing on the health problems such as the deaths from tetanus and sepsis, infertility and chronic infection. If I hadn't then people in my country would have been even more offended and they wouldn't have listened. I remind them that all I want – all anybody wants – is a healthy child. 'I am honour-bound to speak out,' I say. 'You trust me to deliver your children and now you must trust me on this. If a snake was sliding towards your child then I would be failing in my responsibility if I didn't stop it.' I don't give anyone the chance to accuse me of being crude or critical of our culture. I speak only as a medical professional. Women's rights have their place, but not on my battlefield. I don't want to overload the camel.

I believe in my heart that my father would have approved of

what I have done. His sole concern was for his patients, and he too must have had to deal with unnecessary infant mortality and the deaths of otherwise healthy women. He'd have done anything to save those in his care and he was never shy in expressing his opinion or encouraging me to. It is in his memory that I continue to fight against such barbarism and I like to think that, somewhere, he is smiling and nodding.

My mother, on the other hand, was the opposite. I don't think she ever forgave me for shaming her so publicly with such an outspoken campaign. Of all the terrible things I had done in her eyes, this was by far the worst and I was never able to convince her otherwise. It also ended my second marriage, because Bulbul had never expected that beyond my first speech the subject would become my daily occupation as I organized the newly formed committee, developed guidelines, explanations and strategies. My marriage ended in divorce less than a year after I became Director of Health Services. Even though Bulbul had supported my initial efforts to bring the issue under public scrutiny, he resented how much time I devoted to the follow-up conferences around the globe. It seemed to him that I preferred anything but to stay home and play the role of the traditional Somali wife. I guess he had a point.

When a marriage breaks down in our culture it's always the woman's fault. It is the husband who files for divorce and the husband who is allowed to do and say whatever he likes. The wife is just expected to put up with it. In truth, I have not been dealt a good hand in my marriages. This one lasted four years and all attempts at reconciliation and mediation failed to mend the rift between us. My mother was as vocal as ever about my shortcomings. According to her, I should have stayed at home and begged for forgiveness for my many failings. I should never have

given Bulbul cause for suspicion or been so much trouble, and
so on. She didn't understand why I might not want to remain in
a marriage that wasn't working and made me so unhappy. The
embarrassment of being divorced for a second time would, she said,
heap further shame on the whole family. Neither she or Bulbul
understood that if a woman is a professional with her own means
of support, her career should be considered just as important as
her husband's. It never was.

When Bulbul and I decided that enough was enough and the
divorce proceedings began, he went back to one of his previous
wives (just as Mohamed had), my mother moved back to her old
house, and I found myself an apartment. I was done with men,
I told myself. I would never, ever marry again.

CHAPTER SIXTEEN

Muscat, Oman, 1978

Despite my solemn vow, Hassan Kayd was probably always destined to become my third husband. Our paths had been crossing since the 1940s and I guess we had unfinished business. We'd grown up together as children, kicking a ball of rags around the streets of Hargeisa. I'd watched him graduate at Sandhurst. I'd saved his life after the coup in 1961. I'd wept openly when he was arrested and imprisoned, and I'd been reminded of his charm when I visited the north recently.

After my marriage was over and I'd moved into my apartment, Hassan Kayd turned up at my door one day and said, simply, 'Hello, Edna.' When the Ogaden War ended, there was little news of who was alive, who was wounded or who was still missing. My brother had returned skinny, bearded, with long hair and his clothes in tatters, but I had no idea where Hassan was. Seeing him alive made my heart miss a beat and I knew that I was in danger once more. I couldn't help myself. I missed having a husband. I longed for companionship. I hoped with each man I married that they would be different; that they'd understand that a marriage is a partnership and not just the ownership of a woman by a man. I hoped that Hassan, of all people, would finally give me the respect I felt I deserved.

We were married in 1978 at a time of further political upheaval in our country following another failed military coup – this time by officers from the Majeerteen clan who wanted to topple Siad Barre. Soon afterwards Barre summoned Hassan to see him in the middle of the night. The President Boots was an insomniac who conducted many of his meetings in the early hours. Being summoned then meant only two things – imprisonment or promotion. As Hassan left in a sinister-looking government car I had no idea when, or if, I'd ever see him again. I waited up all night to find out. When he returned at 3 a.m., he immediately broke down with the stress.

'What happened?'

'I'm to be appointed the new Somali ambassador to Oman.'

'What? Where? Oman? Where is that?' I had to look it up. Then I asked, 'What gave him that idea?' I knew he had appointed Mohamed ambassador to India only to arrest him again. Was this a similar tactic to send Hassan to jail?

'The Sultan went to Sandhurst too and they want me to foster the relationship between our two countries.' The regime had done its homework.

'Okay, so when do you start?'

'As soon as my credentials are accepted in a month or so.'

Thinking of my important job in the Ministry, I took a deep breath and asked quietly, 'Do you want to go alone?'

He looked horrified and cried, 'No, no, Edna!' Then he said the magic words: 'I need you!'

'But what about my work?'

'You can always come back periodically, and you could maybe manage some of it from there?'

Neither of us then knew that diplomatic protocol dictated otherwise. As the ambassador's wife, it was made quite clear that

I would be expected to move to Muscat with him as an accessory, and also to give up my career. Nobody knew whether I'd agree to such a step, but in the end I did, chiefly because I cared for Hassan and wanted to look after him the best I could. I was also nervous about what might happen to me if I stayed in Somalia. Mohamed Egal was back under house arrest in Mogadishu and I feared for his safety and for his sanity, as I knew how hard it would be, psychologically, to face another loss of liberty.

Although I was determined to make my third marriage more of a success than my previous two, the challenges were enormous from the start. I liked Oman but I was immediately bored because I wasn't allowed to do any paid or even unpaid work there. The idea of not going to work at my department in the ministry or putting on my uniform each day and helping to deliver babies or train nurses was unthinkable to me. I tried to keep from going crazy by playing bridge, collecting seashells and stamps, but that didn't work. In the company of other diplomatic or expatriate wives also forbidden from working I took up golf, jam-making and origami.

Needless to say, when the WHO asked me to speak about FGM and maternal mortality in Sudan and Senegal, I jumped at the chance. I had two long absences from Oman after that. One was in 1982 as a WHO consultant working to convince the government of Djibouti to support a training programme in midwifery. Since Hassan didn't approve of me accepting the two-year contract I was offered, I found a way to complete that consultancy in just eight months. Then in 1983, I accepted a USAID scholarship in New York for four months with Planned Parenthood to study family planning and also learn about the explosion of the new disease of HIV/AIDS that was ravaging the homosexual community.

It was a fascinating time but the most important thing that

happened in America was the rekindling of my dream to build a hospital. I was in my mid-forties and I was starting to have the feeling that time was running out. When I was sent to an outreach project in Harlem, it resurrected my dream. I longed to build a hospital – not for my father this time but a small maternity facility where I could train midwives and showcase the best of healthcare, just like the ones I'd visited in New York. Upon my return to Oman, and with the help of a Swiss architect friend of my brother's who frequently joined us for lunch, I drew up some plans based on what I wanted to cherry-pick from all the best hospitals I had worked in, coupled with my experiences designing the maternity wing at Medina, and then I put them to one side.

I hardly ever went back home during this period, as the news there was increasingly grim. When the 1978 coup failed and its plotters were executed, Barre's generals cruelly punished the clan from which the coup's leader had come. Some 2,000 elders were rounded up and killed, hundreds of women raped, and the nomads' wells and reservoirs destroyed, causing famine on a biblical scale. My brother was one of the many dissidents who publicly opposed Barre after the failure of the Ogaden War cost Somaliland so much of our territory. Fearing that Farah was too obvious a target for arrest, imprisonment and possibly torture, I invited him to visit me in Oman. 'Just stay for a few weeks until things calm down,' I pleaded. He came and never left, resettling in Muscat with his family and working as an engineer with the Oman Mining Company. I was so relieved that he was safe.

In Hargeisa a group of young doctors, teachers and other educated Somalilanders formed a union to try to improve conditions and fix the government hospital, which had deteriorated so badly that there weren't even any doors on the women's toilets. They asked for my help and – if I'd lived there – I would undoubtedly have joined their ranks. Tragically for them, their action was considered subversive by the government and they were arrested and sentenced first to death and then to life imprisonment for 'insulting the revolution' by telling the world that the regime was inefficient. They each served between seven and eight years, much of it in solitary confinement or on death row.

In such a climate, I knew that as long as Siad Barre was in power I would never be allowed to build a hospital, especially as the capital of former Somaliland was the seat of growing dissent. I realized that my hospital would have to be in Mogadishu, if at all. I still didn't know where or how.

Hassan Kayd's term as ambassador ended in 1984 and life for me back in the Somali capital wasn't easy. I had spent the prime years of my life in the city. My first married home had been there; my time as First Lady began there; and I took up my first Ministry directorship there. But Mogadishu was also the place where I'd experienced house arrest and detention, suffered endless harassment and humiliation from the government at work and in my private life, and witnessed the brutality of Barre and his men for the first time. I therefore had very mixed feelings about the city and the memories it left with me.

Unless I chose to defect and take my relatives with me, I knew that I had no choice but to stay there, so I decided to go ahead with my hospital plan. I wanted something good to come out of my experience as a nurse for more than twenty years, midwife and trainer, so I applied for a licence from the Ministry of Health. I was prepared to cash in some of my savings to pay for land and start construction but I needed the government to grant me a site suitable for a hospital. They eventually did – a shabby plot of scrubland next to a site earmarked for a new prison. It cost me $45,000 and was seven kilometres outside the city, but it was all

I could afford. The total area of 15,000 square metres, was lower than the neighbouring plots, so my first challenge was to find enough landfill to level it. From that day on, I would quite literally chase after dumper trucks and tractors in my little Volkswagen, honking my car horn and calling out to the drivers, 'Hey! Stop, stop! Listen, I have some land to fill, do you have time to follow me?' People would often tell me, 'I saw you yesterday, Edna. It looked like you were being chased down the road by a tractor!' It became sort of a joke, but that's how I got the land filled.

Then we built a wall around what I had planned as a two-storey building with sixty to one hundred beds. We brought in water and electricity and started laying roads and driveways. I had my photograph taken standing proudly in front of the hundred stauncheons erected around the concrete foundation slab. It cost me well over $150,000 of my own money to lay the infrastructure and pay for all the materials that I needed before my funds ran out, but for lots of complicated political and other reasons my hospital was never built. My first big problem came when an armed policeman squatted on the land and refused to leave. In the end I had to get the Minister of the Interior to intervene and order him away. I learned later that the guard's presence was part of a crude plot by some individuals and a relative to make me give up the land in order that they could take it for themselves. Some time later, I also discovered that the Sultan of Oman, to whom I had written to ask for support, had donated funds to my hospital but neither the funds nor the information was ever passed on to me. The betrayal cut very deep and the stresses were the death knell for my third marriage.

It is fair to say that I reached the lowest point of my life then. I was broke and a divorcee three times over. I kept asking myself, 'What's wrong with me? Am I such a terrible person?' Eventually,

I decided that I just wasn't the right kind of wife. The truth was that I challenged these husbands of mine. I voiced my own opinions. I mixed and worked with men and women indiscriminately. I thought nothing of leaving my marital bed for an emergency when I wasn't even on night duty. In their eyes, I was a freak and yet, to my mind, I was simply doing my duty with the utmost dedication as I was trained to do, and had witnessed my own father doing all his life. I was his shadow and his mimic. My father was a good 'healer', and I was a good nurse and midwife. Ironically, my husbands' complaints were the same as those I'd heard from my mother throughout my childhood. It made me come to the conclusion that perhaps my father and I had both been impossible to live with.

For the first time in my life I lost all confidence in myself, and in my ability to handle men and money. I felt like ever since Dad died I'd bent over backwards to keep my family off the streets. From the age of fifteen I had never stopped studying or working to the point that I had no time to develop any close friendships, which left me without any personal support. I was even beginning to have serious doubts about my career. My hospital dream had used up all my money and my energy. I didn't have a job as I'd resigned from my position in the civil service to follow Hassan Kayd to Oman. I often had to ask my mother for money for fuel and cigarettes. Without the Sultan's contribution, finishing my project seemed like an impossible fairytale, but what could I do instead? In my lowest moments, I wondered what I had to live for. With almost clinical detachment, I decided that maybe the best way to end my misery would be to drive my Beetle off the cliffs at the end of the old Post Office Road and put an end to it all. Thankfully, Fate had other plans for me.

In the midst of my despair, I applied for a job with the Somali

Red Crescent Society – part of the International Red Cross –
which I had helped found in 1963. The pay was minimal and
I was debating whether I could afford the commute when a telex
arrived out of the blue from the WHO Regional Office for the
Eastern Mediterranean, based in Egypt. It was a gift from the
heavens:

URGENTLY SEEKING YOUR AVAILABILITY AS REGIONAL ADVISOR ON NURSING AND MIDWIFERY FOR THE EASTERN MEDITERRANEAN REGION

After almost begging for a job – any job – I now had an offer of
what seemed like the ideal position for me: a platform to educate
African and Middle Eastern countries on the subjects closest to
my heart. It was with relief and delight that I accepted the position
that would pay me almost $9,000 a month and help me finish
my hospital. In May 1986, I returned to the WHO as regional
advisor based in Alexandria. I arrived in Alexandria with $30 in
my pocket, but was immediately entitled to a $1,000 advance.
That felt to me like a million dollars.

Overnight, and in another abrupt change of fortune, I found
myself responsible for the health and welfare of women and nurses
in twenty-two member states – Afghanistan, Bahrain, Djibouti,
Egypt, Iran, Iraq, Jordan, Kuwait, Lebanon, Libya, Morocco,
Oman, Pakistan, Qatar, Saudi Arabia, Somalia, Sudan, Syria,
Tunisia, United Arab Emirates, Cyprus and Yemen. Over the next
few years I visited most of them on a rotation of eleven countries
per year. I was also in charge of the nursing scholarships to be
distributed to the most qualified students from each country, and
suddenly understood what it must have been like for Miss Udell
from the British Colonial Office. I was so excited to become the

advocate for best practices in midwifery and nursing care over such a vast region, and to be helping to implement them too. I couldn't wait to get started.

***

Over the next five years my travels for the WHO took me from Cairo to Khartoum, Rabat to Karachi, Yemen to Kabul, and beyond. Healthcare had changed massively since I'd been a student and I was eager to share these technological developments wherever I could. The best of all was the Doppler foetal monitor, which was far superior to placing my ear on a mother's belly or listening through an ear trumpet (so often stolen from my car by mischievous children). Most important of all, though, was how far we'd come in terms of hygiene, and the prevention and control of infection with the use of antibiotics.

There were still so many who needed to be educated, though. In Darfur in the Sudan, I was shocked by the incompetence of the trainee midwives I visited. Their fingernails were uncut and blackened with dirt and they took little care of their equipment. I was furious at their laziness, but knew I had to temper my feelings. I did, however, immediately report back that they were a danger to their patients and needed further intensive training.

In the last small village I visited, I met a middle-aged midwife who had a huge swelling on her neck of the thyroid gland, known as goitre. I'm sure she thought that I'd be put off by her deformity as she sat in her little mud hut waiting to meet me, but what struck me most was how clean her equipment was and how utterly professional she was in her treatment of patients. I was so moved by the quiet competence and dedication of this simple woman in the middle of nowhere with scant support and no recognition, that I continue to hold her up as a model for my student midwives. As I was leaving, I handed her $30 as a gift 'from one midwife to another', and she in turn gave me a woven basket, probably the most precious thing she possessed. I later cleaned out all the kernels and hung her generous gift on my office wall, where it remains today. My encounter with her remains more vivid in my memory than all the official dinners and banquets I had to attend in my twenty years with WHO.

The news from Somalia became more and more distressing to hear. Barre had started nothing short of civil war against his own people and was pounding former British Somaliland to dust. International observers are still finding mass graves from that dark time. They contain the bodies of men, women and children who came from the same clans or villages as those opposing Barre. Thousands fled, many to Egypt, and brought with them unbearable stories and even photographs of rape, torture and oppression as thugs went from house to house taking whatever they liked. Although my immediate family was safely out of harm's way, the plight of my people burned deep into my heart and – as their former First Lady – I wanted to do anything I could to help.

In 1988 I agreed to visit Hargeisa for a three-day visit under armed escort to monitor a nursing and maternal health project. My arrival coincided with the beginning of the so-called 'Hargeisa Holocaust', the systematic massacre of people from my clan, in which between 50,000 and 200,000 people were slaughtered over a period of two years, including many of my cousins. The dictatorship created a special unit of the Somali Armed Forces known as *Dabar Goynta Isaak* or the Isaaq Exterminators to do their dirty work. They also planted between one and two million unmarked landmines, booby traps and other lethal devices, predominantly in Isaaq areas.

Less than twelve hours after being back in my tense home

town, I received a message that UNICEF needed to evacuate me urgently because they'd heard that I was under surveillance as an 'anti-revolutionary' and about to be arrested. Despite my high profile and UN credentials, Siad Barre's government still considered me a domestic enemy, particularly since my Isaaq clansmen were leading the rebellion against him. I had no choice but to pack my bag and leave my hotel in the dark at 5 a.m. to fly back to Egypt via Mogadishu.

Within a year, Hargeisa was blockaded and a million people fled to refugee camps in Ethiopia or beyond, many being strafed by machine gun fire from planes overhead. In what was later described as the fastest forced movement of people in Africa, they created the world's largest refugee camp at Harta Sheikh. The few pockets of civilians left behind were brutally punished each time a government soldier was killed or injured. Twenty or so of them would be rounded up and taken to Salaanta – the old parade ground where the 21 October celebrations used to take place – to be flogged and hung or shot. They might be left hanging there for days with signs around their necks accusing them of membership of rebel groups, as a warning to others. In the ensuing months, ninety per cent of Hargeisa would be reduced to rubble by constant aerial and ground bombardment. Burao suffered a similar fate, with seventy per cent destroyed. These atrocities became known as 'the forgotten genocide' in what the reporting organization American Human Rights Watch described as 'a government at war with its own people'.

The healthiest citizens, especially children and teenagers, were forced to donate blood for the Somali Army until they were literally bled dry and their hearts stopped. Soldiers would march into the classrooms and order the children to stand up so that they could pick the tallest and healthiest. Mothers, hearing this, begged their children to crouch or make themselves appear smaller if the soldiers ever marched into their school. Many children died this way and their drained bodies are only now being unearthed from the mass graves found near their schools. Others crawled home to warn their families and friends.

★★★

In spite of the horrific stories from Somalia, in 1988 I agreed to go back to Mogadishu again briefly for the WHO. My visit was shortly before the Jasiira beach massacre of forty-seven Isaaq professionals who were rounded up from their homes at midnight and executed on the communal beach west of the city. As with all these crimes, no one might have known what had happened to them but for one who miraculously survived to tell the story. Although many Isaaqs in Mogadishu had also been detained, the feeling was that the sheer number of foreign, diplomatic and UN staff in the city would make it safer for me to be there. Many of them were living in an exclusive residential district protected by the highest security where a hotel room could cost $500 per night. It amused me to discover that this was on the site of the former Halane boot camp where I had spent four months being indoctrinated into scientific socialism and marching to the beat of Siad Barre's drum.

While in Mogadishu I hoped to check on my land and visit my hospital construction site, which I'd continued to fund in my absence. The city felt extremely tense on my arrival and I agreed to stay with my UN colleagues rather than with relatives to avoid putting them at risk. Despite all our precautions, word got out that I was in the city and two of my uncles found me and begged me to help find a relative, Mohamoud Ahmed, who had been taken to the Digfer hospital as a casualty. Private citizens were forbidden from entering Digfer so they hoped that, as a UN official, I might be able to get in.

I didn't hesitate and went very early the next morning, against all official advice. The place was barely recognizable to me from the time I taught midwives there as the Prime Minister's wife. Just as in Jigjiga, the stench was awful and the floor was covered with bodies, both the dead and seriously wounded in bloodstained clothes. Holding my hand to my mouth and batting away flies, I had to step over stinking, bearded corpses in the search for my missing relative. I had all but given up hope when I heard a voice call, 'Edna!' and there among the others was sixty-year-old Mohamoud, his beard and hair matted with sweat, his hand smashed and bloody. His elbow and wrist were badly twisted and he was in a terrible state.

With the help of a soldier, I managed to get him up and took him by taxi to my mother's house where my cousins were living. I was glad to have been able to save him, though I will never forget the horror of what I witnessed that day. That was the last time I was in Mogadishu and I have never been back to any part of former Italian Somalia since. The land on which I'd hoped to build my hospital was eventually snatched by one of Somalia's many warlords. My deeds and legal documents were no match for guns. My dream was lost. Perhaps that was the plan all along – another way of getting back at Edna Adan Ismail.

★★★

I had never been one to say no to the UN and the important work they were doing, especially at that difficult time when the whole world felt to be at war and I seemed to be living and working in the crucible of conflict.

In early 1989, I agreed to go to Kabul, Afghanistan, as the Russian forces were pulling out after nine years of an abortive Soviet-Afghan War. An estimated two million civilians and over one hundred thousand combatants had been killed, three million were wounded, and millions of Afghanis were displaced or became refugees. Being sent to Kabul proved to be one of my most dangerous UN missions, even though I was assured that I'd be supervised and safe in the UN guest headquarters. What I found when I arrived was quite different. Planes were flying overhead constantly and every four minutes they'd release flares to deter heat-seeking missiles. Curfews from 4 p.m. restricted our movements in most parts of the city. The day before I was to fly out after a nine-day stint, eighteen rockets fell on the city, killing civilians and children. We were lucky they didn't fall on us, but one destroyed a hangar at the airport and set it alight, making us fear that we might not be able to get out.

Expecting casualties, I hurried to inspect the UN dispensary and was shocked to discover that it was completely unprepared for trauma cases or critical emergencies. The mostly bare shelves had eardrops and nose drops, allergy tablets, aspirins, sticking plasters and laxatives. There was no morphine or antibiotics, no bandages, IV fluids, dressings, splints, sutures or surgical instruments. None of that had even been ordered – in a war zone. The man in charge was left in no doubt how angry I was. 'Can you hear those explosions?' I told him. 'Do you have any idea what that means? Have you ever seen someone brought in bleeding to death, or their bodies peppered with shrapnel wounds? If our compound is hit, lives will be lost not because of the bombing but because of the lack of appropriate emergency first aid and management of their condition. People don't die of earache or constipation, they die from the wounds caused by bullets and bombs!'

Before we were eventually evacuated to safety, I made him draw up a list of everything that was needed and I took it with me. On my way home, via India, I burst in unannounced to the UN Office of Logistics Support in New Delhi and gave them the list of emergency supplies that were urgently needed in Kabul. Then I gave them a piece of my mind.

★★★

I was in Alexandria in January 1991 when I heard news from my friends at the Kenyan and Djibouti embassies that the Somali civil war had taken a dramatic turn. A coalition of opposing clans had overthrown Siad Barre who'd fled from Mogadishu in a tank to his clan's stronghold in the southwestern Gedo region. His military dictatorship had been toppled and the Somali National Army disbanded. All UN staff had been evacuated from Mogadishu and were giving security briefings about what was happening there.

At least seven rival militia groups had led the rebellion and, the moment Barre was gone, they began competing for influence in the power vacuum he left. Although he returned to try to seize back control, he was repelled and forced into exile first to Kenya and then to Nigeria. A few years later he died of a heart attack in Lagos while sitting on his toilet. Sadly for the people of Somalia three decades later they haven't yet found a leader to take their country out of the situation that is often described as 'the world's worst failed state'. Luckily, Somaliland separated from it.

Barre had done so many terrible things to my country and to my people that it was a blessed relief to see him deposed. He left Somaliland destroyed and traumatized and – almost thirty years later – we are still reeling from the aftershocks. I will, however, begrudgingly give him credit for a few things he did in his twenty-one year dictatorship that I am grateful for. Our language was entirely oral before he came to power, handed on through stories and poems and songs. It was Barre who decided to introduce an official script for the first time, massively increasing literacy. He also gave women like me a platform to speak about women's rights and raised awareness of our role in Somali society. Even though he did all this for his own political reasons, it still gave an example of what could be done. If only he had focused on doing good for the world, instead of all the fighting and cruelty, he could have made a great leader and done so much more for our country. Instead, he will for ever be remembered as a despot and a tyrant, and always to me as General Boots.

Not long after this latest tragic development for Somalia, and when I'd just returned from a conference in Ghana, I was summoned to see my WHO Regional Director who asked me, the moment I entered his office, 'How soon can you go to Djibouti?'

'Why, what happened?' I asked, thinking there must have been an earthquake or some other humanitarian crisis. I was involved in so many important projects at my desk at that time that I was immediately anxious about having to leave them.

'You are to be temporary WHO country representative there for three months,' he told me. 'You'll be stepping into the shoes of the previous Representative who has had to fly to Iraq to arrange his affairs in advance of the expected Gulf War.' Being a WHO country representative was never part of my plan, which was to finish my projects and then take a leave of absence and decide what I wanted to do with the rest of my life. As always, though, I had no choice but to accept my mission, so I parked my car in the garage, packed my bags, locked my apartment and flew to the country where my education had first begun.

My 'temporary' posting which began in March 1991 lasted six-and-a-half years. Not only did the Gulf War break out but there were also major humanitarian crises in Somalia, Yemen, Ethiopia and Eritrea. Refugees flooded into Djibouti and had to be placed in vast camps. The only water they had was dirty and muddy, scraped from the ground and fought over by animals and humans. It made everyone sick. Having toured the Hol Hol camp – which had 30,000 refugees – and seen the problem for myself I told a group of men that I would give them my own money to dig out a proper well deep enough to reach cleaner water. 'I will also provide a fence around it to keep the donkeys out and pipes to transport it, but only if you do the digging first,' I said. Desperate for water, they did as I asked and we soon managed to provide a decent water supply to thousands in that camp. It was so successful that when UNICEF representatives came and saw what I had done they decided to follow suit elsewhere. I also opened a dispensary with nurses to tend to the sick and we set up a disease control centre to deal with parasites, respiratory infections, TB and anaemia. It was the most challenging time of my life but of course I loved it because I was fixing things for the country that had first opened the door to my education.

I'd not long been in my new office when I heard through my diplomatic friends that Mohamed Egal was in extreme danger in Mogadishu. He and several other opposition politicians and prominent people had been under house arrest for several months and were lucky to have escaped execution in the final months of Siad's disintegrating dictatorship. I was astonished that Mohamed hadn't fled to safety after his release from imprisonment in 1985, and was extremely worried about him. Eager to find out more, I learned that he was being held with the Hargeisa shopkeeper who'd greedily demanded fifty dollars from me after my father died. Relying on my contacts in the UN, the Red Cross and my connections to the embassies, including the American ambassador, I immediately appealed on their behalf and managed to get them out on a Red Cross evacuation flight to Djibouti. My priority was Mohamed whom I hardly recognized when we were finally reunited in the hotel we'd checked him into. We hugged and we cried and then we sat and talked. I hadn't seen him in years and was shocked at how thin he was. He had straggly grey hair, an unkempt beard and he stank. His face was gaunt and his sunken eyes looked haunted by what he'd been through. A piece of sticky tape was all that held his broken spectacles together, and his stinking jacket was at least two times too big, giving him the appearance of a scarecrow. I helped clean him up and arranged for him to receive a medical check-up before providing him with some new clothes and glasses. He needed money and a passport, somewhere to live and time to rest.

In spite of how dreadful Mohamed looked, I was extremely relieved to see him and he seemed pleased to see me, too. He was also very grateful because we both knew he would almost certainly have died in Mogadishu if I hadn't been able to get him out. Our emotional reunion gave us the first opportunity to talk face to face since we'd divorced twenty years earlier. Most importantly, we finally had the chance to discuss our marriage and all that had passed between us. We had both felt wronged but admitted that neither of us had tried hard enough to fix our relationship. We were too preoccupied with our own situations, and competing for control. Two decades on we were older and wiser. We not only forgave each other but each felt renewed and healed. I was very happy that we could once again be friends and allies without the burden of a marriage.

Mohamed was too unwell to attend the historic conference in Burao on 18 May 1991 where the clan elders called for
Somaliland's formal separation from the ill-fated union with
Somalia and elected a new interim president. Once he was fully
recovered, Mohamed was offered political asylum by the United
Arab Emirates and he moved there for a while to lick his wounds.
Before he departed he returned to Somaliland to see what he could
do for our beloved country. In Hargeisa he was welcomed as a
hero. As he was driven around the heavily mined streets, he used
the video camera he'd borrowed from me to film the conditions.
It was devastating to see how much of the city had been destroyed.
The house my father had built was in ruins and there was hardly
anything I recognized about our old neighbourhood. There was
little or no infrastructure or medical facilities and, without clean
water, there were cholera epidemics and our people died in their
hundreds.

With so much going on in Somaliland, Djibouti and elsewhere,
the WHO extended my posting to Djibouti and also made me
head of logistics support for Somaliland. As the new head of WHO
I went to see Hargeisa for myself a few months later and found
the experience utterly heartbreaking. I flew in as the leader of a
team of nine, all of them white except for me. We consisted of
two women and seven men who were senior representatives of
various UN Agencies such as UNICEF, UNHCR, the World
Food Programme and UNDP. We were told we'd be met by our
counterparts in Hargeisa on arrival, who were supposed to show
us around. Our little aircraft landed on a very windy morning on
a bumpy runway full of potholes and littered with the detritus of
war, including upturned tanks and broken MIG jets. There was
no sign of any delegation and as there were several local militias
still fighting aggressively for control of the airport, I made sure

that my black face was the first to emerge from the plane. Looking around, I spotted a lone soldier guarding the runway so I raised both my hands and shouted in Somali that I wanted to talk to him.

He strolled over, suspiciously, and asked, 'Who are you?

'I am *Ina Adan Dhakhtar*, Edna Adan Ismail,' I told him with a smile. 'I am from Hargeisa. I am from Somaliland and we are here on a mission to find out the situation on the ground after the war. Is there anybody waiting for us?' He shook his head. 'Then how are we to get into the city?' He shrugged. In an empty lot I spotted an old pick-up and asked whose it was. He gave me the name and I immediately lied and said, 'Oh, that's my uncle. He won't mind me using it!' I asked him to send the driver to me and I then persuaded him to take us the five kilometres into town in return for the price of several tanks of fuel. My female colleague, who was Dutch, sat up front with me, so the other senior UN officials had no choice but to climb up and ride shotgun in the back. The passenger door didn't have hinges and there was no key so the driver started it by sparking two wires together and off we set, keeping to tyre tracks in the dust – the only safe passage through the mines.

I asked the driver to show us what was left of the town so that we could see the damage for ourselves. We found what was left of my father's house and it was just as Mohamed had filmed it, but I couldn't get out of the pick-up because of the mines. Then he took us to meet some Somaliland officials in what was known as 'Morgan's House', as it had been built by Siad Barre's ruthless son-in-law who was known as the 'Butcher of Hargeisa'. When my uncles heard that I was in town, they came to see me and scolded me for taking such a risk in coming as Hargeisa wasn't yet stable. I handed over the $1,000 I'd brought to give them for food – if there was any available in the local market. When we had seen all we could we were taken back to the airport and I reluctantly left my beleaguered city behind.

A few months later I returned with two women, my Dutch colleague and an American. We found the streets of Hargeisa full of 'technicals', open-top vehicles fitted with mortars and anti-aircraft guns. It felt different and more threatening. One of these vehicles began to follow us as soon as I came out of the interim Ministry of Health building. Having seen them in close pursuit, I tapped our driver on the shoulder and told him, 'Stop the car.' He looked at me as if I was insane. 'I said stop this car!' Once we'd pulled over in the dust, I jumped out and confronted our pursuers – four or five men dripping in guns and ammunition.

'Do you think you'll get bigger testicles for shooting Edna Adan in Hargeisa, her home town?' I asked them, scared out of my wits but determined not to show it. 'And do you honestly think you'd get away with it?' By talking their kind of vulgar language and with the help of a crowd that gathered and acted as 'street lawyers' I managed to persuade them to let us on our way. Word soon got out that I was in town and had a lot of money with me so another group of men came after me at my hotel later that night. At 11 p.m. there was banging on my door and a hotel security guard told me that there were militias outside threatening to blow up the building if I, Edna, didn't come down to the lobby.

'And you expect me to come out?' I asked through the locked and bolted door, adding, 'Who are they anyway?'

'I don't know, but they have a tank.'

'You mean a military tank? Just a minute, hold on.' I found a pen and a piece of paper and slid it under the door and told him to ask them to write down what they wanted with me. The paper came back with the message that they wanted money and to be hired by me. I turned the paper around and wrote: 'Thank you for your visit but there is no way I get out of my bed for anyone. I am sure, as Somali gentlemen, you have brought me the traditional *sooryo* gifts offered to a visiting woman and I am very happy that you have, as I've spent all my money and don't know how I am going to pay my hotel bill tomorrow. Instead of a gift, could you please settle it for me? Thank you very much, Edna Adan Ismail.'

I never heard another word but the following morning I asked the guard what they'd said when he showed them my note. He said, 'They just laughed and went away.'

Knowing that law and order had to be restored as soon as possible, before I left Hargeisa the next day I went to see the city's general hospital where I had first worked as a qualified nurse back in Somaliland, a building that was now in such a sad state of repair that I almost wept. If ever a new hospital was needed, it was there – in my hometown – and yet I was no longer in the position or the mindset to undertake such a major project.

That visit above all else convinced me that my country needed strong leadership to bring some semblance of order. We finally got it in May 1993 when Mohamed Egal attended another reconciliation conference – this time in Borama – and was almost unanimously elected President of Somaliland. I couldn't imagine a better man for the job. While thousands of tons of UN humanitarian aid was being airlifted into Somalia under 'Operation Provide Relief' and 'Operation Restore Hope' to help the estimated three million starving, our northern part of the country received very little and it was clear that a formal and legal separation from war-torn Somalia had to be orchestrated urgently.

Almost immediately, Mohamed began to write to me in Djibouti begging me to come home and help him. It wasn't a romantic proposition – he had married again – but a political one. 'Our country needs so much but it needs its "Mother Edna" more than ever,' he'd tell me. Each time I flew into Hargeisa, he'd send a car to pick me up from the terminal, which had been renamed Egal Airport in his honour. He also gave me a bodyguard to escort me around town and to his home for lunch with him and his wife, who I'm sure found it odd having to entertain his ex-wife in her home. Just as we had when we were married, Mohamed and I bounced ideas off each other and endlessly discussed the political situation long after his wife had left the table. More than ever before, we were able to talk frankly and openly and I valued his counsel as much as he valued mine. He would try out new ideas on me and I'd react to them. I might say, 'Fantastic', or – more often than not – 'No, no, no, that won't work. Why don't you try this... ?'

In my spare time I'd drive to my father's house and survey the ruins of the place he'd been so proud of, which only made me more nostalgic for the old days. The entire area of our neighbour-hood was strewn with landmines and every building had been ransacked. All that was left of the family home was part of a wall with a single window frame and the split trunk of an acacia tree my parents used to sit under for shade. Nothing else. The looters had taken everything. I managed to salvage a cut stone from the front of the old house. So many sad and fond memories.

I was incredibly torn about the idea of returning to Somaliland one day. I was fifty-six years old and would have to retire from the WHO at sixty under its compulsory rules, but what then? There was nothing but rubble for me to come back to in Hargeisa and the prospect of years of heartache, conflict and deprivation. My brother Farah was still in Oman with his family, and my mother and sister had made a new life for themselves in England with my nieces and nephews – all of whom I had delivered myself and thought of as my surrogate children. Longing to be closer to them

I visited London and was leaning towards retiring there when I was told by an acquaintance about a reasonably priced, fully-furnished apartment for sale not far from my mother in Wembley. It seemed perfect for me so I paid the deposit and agreed to wire the rest of the asking price once I returned to Djibouti.

Fate intervened once more, though, with the events of the Battle of Mogadishu in October 1993, graphically depicted in the Hollywood movie *Black Hawk Down*. A team of 160 US special servicemen was sent in to capture the leaders of the Habr Gidr clan of the self-proclaimed Somali leader Mohamed Farrah Aidid. It was supposed to be a lightning strike but Aidid's men shot down two Black Hawk helicopters and damaged two others. As a result, the entire world, including me, was shocked to see the television footage showing the body of the American marine mutilated and dragged through the streets of Mogadishu. The subsequent task force sent in to rescue the beleaguered crews sparked a fierce battle in which approximately one thousand civilians and combatants died, including eighteen American soldiers. Hundreds more were wounded. The news shocked the world, and by the time I heard it back in Djibouti I too was shattered.

That was when the estate agent in London contacted me to tell me that the sale of the apartment had fallen through. 'What? Why?' I asked.

'The vendor says he couldn't possibly sell his property to a Somali.'

No matter how much I protested there was nothing I could do. People the world over have always found it difficult to separate Somaliland from Somalia – the world's most lawless state run by warlords with the highest piracy rate. For years there have been calls that we should change our name to something that sounds completely different. One suggestion is Mayland, as all the great things that have happened to our country historically happened in the month of May, a time of rain and plenty. My favourite suggestion, though, is Gollisia after the Gollis range of mountains that runs from east to west across every part of our nation. In truth, even 'Camelland' would be better than any connection to Somalia.

The misunderstanding by the flat owner in London finally hardened my resolve to return to my homeland and rebuild my life there. If nothing else I wanted to help show the world that Somaliland was decidedly NOT Somalia.

CHAPTER SEVENTEEN

Hargeisa, Somaliland, 1993–1996

Before I moved back to my country for good and began to think seriously about maybe building my maternity hospital there, I had some unfinished business to attend to. As the eldest child of Adan Doctor Ismail I knew that it was my duty to rebuild my father's house. It would have been seen as disrespectful and irresponsible if I'd dared undertake anything else while his property stood in ruins. People would have accosted me in the street and told me, 'Have you no shame, Edna? Look at your family house!'

Flying in and out of Hargeisa from Djibouti, I witnessed the incredibly courageous work of the international teams as they cleared entire areas of landmines and other ordnance. I also saw how homeless families followed the mine-clearers and immediately squatted on any land that had been made safe. My father's plot was no exception and on one of my visits I found unfamiliar kids running around in the rubble-strewn yard. When I informed the squatters that this was private land, one told me, 'The fathers of these children died liberating this country. They have a right to live here. If you are coming back to live in it, we will move out. We know this land is not a carpet; we will not roll it up and take it with us. But if you are not going to live in it, then these children must stay.' I explained that I had to respect my promise to my broken family to rebuild our broken house and that it was my intention to live on the property. Naturally, I paid them to go.

With the agreement of my brother and sister that I should hire a contractor and start construction as soon as possible, I set about designing it. Instead of replicating what my father had done in the 1950s, I decided to make it a large modern two-storey house – the likes of which had never been seen in Hargeisa before. I wanted it to be an example to other Somalis that now was a good time to come back and invest in Somaliland. The biggest problem was finding experienced builders and artisans. Many had died in the war and many more fled to Saudi Arabia or the Emirates where their skills could bring them a higher salary. Others had lost limbs and had to beg simply to survive. Even when we found workmen, we had to ship in supplies from Dubai. Before we could even begin construction we needed to bulldoze away a metre of topsoil to make certain there were no unexploded landmines lurking. With all these problems it took three years before the property was finished, but the experience taught me some invaluable lessons about construction. I oversaw every phase and learned where to find a good mason, how much to pay a carpenter, and where to haggle for the best deal on concrete. The resulting property was considered such an oddity when it was done that people came and took photographs of it and of me – 'crazy Edna' rebuilding her father's house in a time of war. 'Why is she building a palace in the ruins?' I'd hear them say. 'She's lost her mind.' I'm only grateful that my mother was far away in London and too mentally absent with dementia by then to know what people were saying about me now.

The United Nations Development Program (UNDP) rented my completed house from me as soon as it was ready in 1996, which helped supplement my small UN pension once it kicked in. My hospital would eventually rise brick by brick with my own money, but it was important for my family and for our community that I had done my duty first – Doctor Adan's house had been restored.

Every day I was in Hargeisa my father was never far from my thoughts. The city was my umbilical cord to him. I remembered those times when he'd return after several days of treating nomads in the bush – the first time I ever spotted grey in his hair. He'd be tired, dusty and unshaven – but rather than coming straight home, he would always stop by his hospital first. I also thought of how many times I'd helped him roll up bandages or clean up the treatment room as he told me wistfully, 'I wish I had better facilities than this, Shukri', or mused, 'If only I had good instruments to work with.' Much as I still missed him, I was grateful at least that he wasn't alive to witness the destruction of our country or see the state his hospital was in now. It was filthy and broken without any piped water and squatters with their donkeys and goats living in the grounds. Some were even keeping their animals in the wards and I took a photograph of goats nibbling at a patient's blankets. All the midwives had left or been killed, lost limbs or were in refugee camps, so the only people delivering babies were the traditional birth attendants with all their inexperience and bad habits. The women of my city deserved a far better quality of care.

The more time I spent in Hargeisa, the more my resolve to fulfil my childhood dream strengthened. It was clearer than ever to me that building my father a hospital in Somaliland was what I had been working towards my whole life. The plans had been floating around in my head so long that it was finally time to put all that I had learned and experienced into practice – in his name. Now, I just had to figure out how, where and with what.

★★★

My first challenge was to find a piece of land. Mohamed was the obvious place to start but even he thought I was mad. 'What do you mean you want to build a hospital? Can't you get hospitals out of your system? Haven't you had enough of them? What about your retirement, Edna? Why don't you just relax like anyone else? You're not a young woman any more.'

Squaring up to him, I replied, 'Now more than ever I have to do this because all our health facilities have been destroyed by war. Surely, you can understand that or do you like being the President of a country with no decent hospitals?' I watched him squirm.

'Well, what do you want from me?'

'First of all, I want your blessing, and then I want the government's permission to build a hospital. I don't want to have to jump through as many hoops again as I did with Siad Barre in Mogadishu.' President Egal not only gave me his blessing and his permission, he then offered to help me find a plot of land somewhere on the outskirts of Hargeisa. My initial reaction was that the edge of town would be the wrong location. Women who go into labour at all hours of the day and night need an easily accessible facility not one in the middle of nowhere. I told him, 'Our women are not lepers who need to be sent out to a quarantine, Mohamed. They need a place they can get to quickly when their labour starts. It must also be big enough to expand as our needs grow.' I wanted a site big enough to accommodate all the dreams I'd been carrying in my head.

After a long period of reflection and discussion, Mohamed only had bad news for me. 'The town has no vacant space large enough for your hospital except... well, except *that place*.'

I recoiled. I knew exactly where he meant. *That place* was Salaanta, the old military parade ground where Siad Barre and his generals used to proudly parade their military hardware and weapons of destruction and death. As opposition to his regime had intensified, it then became the place where government security forces would round up dissidents and publicly punish them – often by execution. Not surprisingly it was regarded as a hated place, even a haunted one. Avoided by all, it was turned into a communal dump where residents threw all their household garbage, old tyres, even the carcasses of dead donkeys. Since the civil war and the expansion of a nearby squatters' camp for 15,000 displaced people it became a no-man's land – dirty, smelly, neglected and despised. People used to say, I live beyond *that place*, or I am walking in the direction of *that place*… everyone knew what *that place* meant. The suggestion that I should build my gleaming new hospital there offended me deeply. Furious, I told him, 'That is a place where people died, Mohamed! I want to build you a place where people live. It is a hospital – a facility that has to be clean. You don't build a hospital on a place that's haunted by the souls of the murdered. I can't build it on a dirty, infected, smelly piece of land!'

My fury rising, I jumped up and wagged a finger at him. 'You men will never understand! It is because I want to build a hospital for women that you made this offensive suggestion.' I turned and stomped out of his office. Still seething inside, I flew back to Djibouti the next day, ready to give up my dream, move to London and look for a teaching job. I told myself that I would have to completely rethink my life, but not in Africa. 'They took my home, my husband, my life, and now they won't let me build my hospital?' I yelled at the walls. I decided it was time to leave and to move on without the hospital in my head for the first time in fifty years.

The more I thought about what my life would be like without my dream, and about how much good I could do with my own healthcare facility, the more the hospital won – every time. If it took accepting the only land that was on offer, then maybe that is what I would have to do. I then began to wonder if maybe *that place* wasn't such a bad idea after all. Perhaps the site south of the river in a poor section of town that never had a hospital before was exactly where I should build a hospital. If a woman from that area was sick or had a pregnancy complication and needed medical attention, she would have to walk four kilometres to get to the Group Hospital, as there was no public transport and no bridges across the river. If there were a flood then she'd have to wait for the waters to abate, by which time she and her baby would probably be dead. It was in the poorest quarters that the gruesome statistics of maternal mortality from eclampsia, infection, a ruptured uterus, haemorrhage, disease and sepsis were the highest. Maybe it wasn't such a ridiculous suggestion after all to build a hospital on a place that had known injustice, pain and suffering and was like a big ulcer in the heart of the city, in an area where there had never been a hospital before. I flew back to Hargeisa secretly contrite – not that I was going to let Mohamed know that.

'Well, do you have any other bright ideas about where this hospital should be?' I began when I met with him again.

He sighed heavily. 'Edna, we talked to the mayor. He agreed that there really is no other available place. If you want to make your hospital smaller, maybe we can find you some other spot nearer the centre of town.'

I shook my head and tutted. 'Come on, Mohamed! A hospital is a small city in itself. I cannot have one without a kitchen or an operating theatre, without in-patient wards or outpatient clinics. A first-rate hospital needs a laboratory, a pharmacy and parking spaces. There is no way that I can make it smaller.'

Mohamed shrugged. 'Then I really don't know what else to

suggest. You can still have that land outside the city – if you want it.'

'Apart from anything else, it's sitting under a mountain of trash,' I complained, wrinkling my nose. 'It's a horrible place where the hungriest people and animals scavenge for food and anything worthwhile. Even if I were to accept it, how would I clear it?'

Sensing a chink in my armour, my first husband smiled. 'Well, if you agree to build there, you won't have to worry about the trash. That's the easiest part. We'll clear it and level the ground for you.' I didn't give him an answer straight away, but as I left his office we both knew that we had struck a deal.

Mohamed kept his word – the authorities bulldozed the 9,600 square metres of land and carted away thirty-two truckloads of trash to burn. The land was levelled and then God sent the rains to wash its past away. I thank God for that and for the fact that Mohamed had his bright idea, because I never would have thought about *that place*. Once again, President Egal proved to be something of a visionary.

★★★

I finally retired from the WHO in September 1997 after a brief stint in Boston studying public health, followed by a debriefing retreat in Geneva to prepare me for retirement. It was at that relaxed gathering of other UN retirees that I heard them all excitedly discussing how they were going to buy a boat, or a house in Spain, move closer to their grandchildren, or take a cruise.

'And what about you, Edna?' they asked.

'Me? Oh, I'm going to go back to my country to build a hospital.'

Their mouths fell open one by one.

I returned to Hargeisa with my belongings in boxes. I cashed in my savings, sold my Mercedes and many of my most valuable possessions, used my retirement payment and money owed for accrued leave, and began to draw my WHO pension. I had estimated the cost of the hospital to be in the region of $400,000 and this is what I used to start its construction. In the end, of course, it was more than double that figure.

I chose to live and work on the construction site every day because I wanted to be part of the crew. I toiled with my labourers, I blistered my hands alongside the brickmakers as we mixed concrete to make bricks in special moulds, and I ate what they ate under the shade of a tree – food prepared by a local woman, Samsam, who cooked for us. I am sure they found me bossy and overbearing but some of the things they disliked most about me were the facts that I prevented them from fighting, chewing khat on my property and carrying weapons. I also hired and trained nine local women to make me 10,000 bricks (which almost caused a walkout as they became our country's first female brickmakers), but the men accepted it in the end, chiefly because I paid them extra. Most of all, though, I think they resented the whistle I hung around my neck. As I couldn't shout as loud as a man, I blew that instead and everyone would turn around to see what I wanted. Pointing, I'd say, 'I need you, the guy in the red shirt. I want to talk with you in my office.'

That first 'office' was a pile of cement blocks under the shade of a single acacia tree. After a few weeks some of the workers took pity on me and built me a small shack from discarded cardboard boxes held together with twigs and string. This was as good as any air-conditioned office I'd occupied in my previous life. Anyone who visited me there would be welcomed into 'Edna's Office'. It was at this time that I started to cover my head with a scarf – not for religious reasons – but because we had no running water and I was tired of combing the brick dust out of my hair.

Over the years, and especially after my construction experiences in Mogadishu, the design of my hospital had evolved gradually. I'd had input from many different people – including architects – and would add something new whenever I had another 'bright idea'. Finally I had what I felt was a reasonable design for a public building in a developing country. It would be on three floors and I had to include everything from a delivery room to a mortuary. Quite apart from having enough space to receive patients, examine them and see them through to a successful birth, I had to think about parking, septic tanks, and the location of the diesel generator as Hargeisa had no electricity and we'd regressed back to paraffin lamps and independent power sources. Once the layout was decided, I hired a crew to dig the foundations. Their first task was to erect a series of small low-rise buildings that would eventually become shops and the pharmacy, but would serve as my first office until I had something better. I oversaw everything from the purchase and transportation of materials in Dubai to the completion of the perimeter wall. As everything I needed was bought with my savings and pension I had a deeply personal interest in making sure that not a shilling was wasted.

At night I slept in a house I shared with my cousin, a deputy bank manager, and his wife, my only other companion a pretty stray cat that adopted me in the street. I called her Shabel, which means Tiger. She wasn't Sanu but she was friendly enough. At sunrise each morning, I'd return to the building site and continue telling the workmen what to do. When the shipload of wood, steel, wires, piping, toilets, paint, washbasins, tiles, shovels, buckets, scaffoldings and cement mixers arrived by ship in Berbera, I hired thirteen trucks and hurried around town buying the rope

and boxes we'd need to shift and store everything. The convoy
that left the port that night was the longest anyone had ever seen,
least of all under the management of a woman. The two-hundred-
kilometre journey took three days. In some places the road was
nothing more than a dirt track. Our convoy frequently had to
stop because one of the trucks had blown a tyre, run out of fuel,
or become bogged down in a riverbed and needed to readjust
its load. We also had to remain vigilant every step of the way to
prevent looting. Since I carried all the receipts to prove that my
goods had made a legitimate entry into Somaliland, I had to drive
ahead of the convoy and show the documents at every checkpoint
(with a bribe I paid only reluctantly), and then hurry to the back
of the convoy to see what was holding up any stragglers and make
sure that nothing was being offloaded.

As my hospital slowly progressed, my biggest concern was
where on earth I would find the staff to work in it once it was
complete. Because we'd trained so many nurses in the past I hoped
and believed that if I advertised I would be able to get them back
from wherever they had fled to, even though I would undoubtedly
have to retrain them all after so many years. To my delight, the
WHO lured me back briefly to consult on the rebuilding of the old
Hargeisa nursing school that was opened in the mid-1960s. It was in
ruins so I worked with an engineer on its redesign, the UNHCR,
the UN Refugee Agency, paid for it to be rebuilt and I banked a
month's salary. Best of all, the school would provide the country
with the qualified staff it needed for government facilities, while
I'd start training those I'd needed for my own hospital. Finding a
doctor was much more of a problem – there were probably only
ten or so (and only two of them obstetricians) in the entire country
with a population of four million. It occurred to me then that, of all
the crazy things I had done, this was the craziest – I was building a

maternity hospital without any obstetrician available to look after my patients. Anywhere else, this would be considered madness, but I reminded myself that it was precisely this shortage of healthcare professionals as well as the lack of hospitals that brought me back to Somaliland in the first place.

I sent out appeals to anyone I thought might be able to help but because of the in-fighting, kidnappings and piracy in neighbouring Somalia foreign doctors were afraid to come, confusing the two countries just as my London vendor had. Then I approached the UN agencies whose staff already worked in Somaliland, but they merely offered to send supplies once my laboratory opened. One senior UNICEF official went further and openly stated that mine was 'an over-ambitious project that could never get completed'. As a belated gesture of goodwill, he sent me buckets, picks and shovels. (Luckily, his replacement gave me some basic supplies and medicines after my hospital was opened and, today, UNICEF is one of our stronger partners.) The buckets and shovels arrived on the day a reporter from the *New York Times* named Ian Fisher visited my construction site after waiting all day to speak to me at an AIDS conference. The article he wrote about me which was published globally (but not in Somaliland) on 29 November 1999 was entitled '*A woman of firsts and her latest feat*'.

Thousands of readers around the world saw the article, including Mayor Richard J. Daley of Chicago, who invited me and a Somali poet named Hadrawi to help the US city mark the new millennium – all expenses paid. It was part of the mayor's Simple Citizens' Millennium Banquet in which two citizens from two hundred countries around the world were selected to attend as guests. When his secretary rang to tell me whom she represented, I thought it was one of my nieces teasing me, so I told her, 'And I'm the Queen of Sheba!' She assured me the offer was genuine and promised to fax me details. By that time I had electricity twice a day thanks to the local baker – a man I'd helped in the past – who kindly strung a wire from his bakery to my office so that I had power whenever he was making bread. Somebody else had donated an old fax machine to me, but the special thermal paper was extremely hard to come by and very expensive. Mayor Daley's secretary kept her word, but overnight, thirty-two pages arrived – needlessly sent twice – for Hadrawi and me. My paper was all used up.

The week in Chicago was certainly something to remember, with an Old Year's Breakfast, tours of the city and a performance of dance from around the world. At the grand banquet I wore my traditional nomadic dress, and then there were fireworks at midnight. When the trip was over, I was flown to Minnesota at the invitation of the Somali community living there, many of whom had fled to the States as refugees. In a theatre crammed with black faces I spotted one white face and immediately took pity on her, as the entire evening was conducted in Somali. For two hours I spoke about what life was like in Somaliland now and answered questions about whether it was safe to return. When the white woman approached me afterwards, I apologized to her for what must have been a boring evening. 'I didn't come to hear you talk, I came to meet you,' she told me. Her name was Sandy Peterson, a travel agent, who had read the *New York Times* article and told me she wanted to help.

'Why, thank you!' I said. 'We need all the help we can get.'

Sandy's one stipulation was that she never donated to any charity unless she had seen it working for herself. True to her word, she flew out to Hargeisa soon afterwards to visit the hospital and see exactly what I was doing, which, at that point, was resurrecting my childhood needlework skills to sew curtains and sheets. She was so impressed that she set up the Friends of Edna Maternity Hospital Charity in the USA enlisting like-minded American men and women who had read the article and made contact with others. Their generous donations became the first lifeline of my hospital and paid for all the windows and doors and much of the flooring. Other donations followed from the Minnesota community, who sent me home from my visit with $2,000 they'd raised at my event, and spoke about me to other Somalis in the US. Most generous of all were the local business people in Somaliland who donated construction materials, cement or cash.

Even better news was that the UNHCR, which had a big refugee population to worry about in Somaliland, had finally agreed to provide me with two doctors and would pay their salaries if I'd agree to cover their food and accommodation and provide a dispensary for the refugees, the UN staff and their families. I agreed instantly. The British embassy in Addis Ababa sent beds, cots, a plastic skeleton, and mannequins for my nurses to train on, all of which are still in use today. While I waited for the UN to send me my doctors, the Edna Adan Hospital quietly opened its outpatients department and laboratory on 23 January 2002. The main building was a long way off completion and my snag list was getting longer as the workmen repeatedly failed to follow my instructions about everything from the location of light switches to why I wanted a window in a particular place.

The young woman Samsam was still cooking for the construction crew on site most days, but one day she didn't turn up for work with their meal. Wondering where she was, and knowing she was pregnant, I made some enquiries and a relative discovered her haemorrhaging at home after a neighbour who'd delivered her baby pulled on the umbilical cord to hasten the placenta. When I heard what had happened, I arranged for her to be taken immediately to the General Hospital and I personally donated blood for the transfusions she needed. She not only survived but her eldest daughter Hamda, then aged eleven, who witnessed her mother's near death, came to train with me as a midwife years later and is now a midwife and chief anaesthetist at my hospital. Life never fails to surprise and reward me.

When my cousin and his wife moved to a smaller house, I had no choice but to give them my cat Shabel and move into an unfinished apartment on the first floor of my hospital, which was eight months away from completion. It has been my home ever since. I had expected to build a small house for myself on site, but as the construction took over my life I couldn't afford to waste the money when I badly needed to finish my hospital. The spot where I'd envisaged my own little house is now the student toilet block and the more I got used to living on site, the better I felt about it. If this place was good enough for my patients then it should be good enough for me. With my budget far exceeded, my funds started to run out and I had to lay off the decorators for six months until my next few pension payments had accrued. People who flocked to the site to watch my progress would ask me, 'Why are you leaving the hospital half painted, Edna?' so I'd tell them the truth: 'I don't have the money.' I'm not sure they believed me. Visiting the crazy old lady who was building a hospital in a ruined country was now a must for anyone flying into Hargeisa, especially foreign aid workers. It was like going to Paris and not visiting the Eiffel Tower.

On another occasion, and in desperation, I went to my brother in Oman and asked him for the last of my valuables which I had kept in his safekeeping. I sold the lot to pay for toilets, taps and washbasins – it was the ultimate in recycling. I figured that I only wore that jewellery occasionally but that now I would use it every single day, along with scores of others who'd be grateful for the facilities my rings and bracelets paid for. I felt truly liberated. The hospital became my home, my office, my everything. There was still no electricity so I lived after dark by the light of the kind of kerosene lamp we'd relied on in my childhood. The smell of the wicks burning transported me straight back to those nights of my father reading by the fire and moths flapping on the fly screens. It took me an age to sort out my belongings from boxes and I confess it was a bit scary, alone there at night in the dead silence but for the occasional barking of a dog. As the plot had once been a killing ground, I half expected ghosts and planned to confront any that might still be hanging around. If they wanted to haunt anybody they had to talk to me first.

The progress of my hospital wasn't just measured in bricks and mortar but in the dedication and support of many people who helped breathe life into my project. Everyone was behind it. Somali neighbours and friends came through for me on numerous occasions when I needed help, a loan or cement. The people from Somaliland Beverage Industries, who run the world's remotest Coca-Cola bottling plant, gave me all the scaffolding I needed, and donated four hundred bags of cement. The municipality gave me fifty truckloads of sand and someone else lent me a truck to transport it. A construction company gave me steel for the top floor and fifty cubic metres of wood, and people who had nothing material to give me offered me free labour. Perhaps most appreciated of all, the people gave me their blessings.

Aside from the wonderful Friends of Edna Maternity Hospital three doctors visited me in the early days from the Tropical Health & Education Trust at King's College Hospital, London. They sat with me under the shade of my tree and asked how they could help. They promised me that they had medical volunteers ready to come when my hospital was finished. I thanked them and promised to be in touch when we were up and running. They kept their word and later sent a team of eleven people for two weeks who were pivotal in getting us started. At around the same time a friend from Somaliland, who was connected to volunteers from an American charity called Hope Worldwide, contacted me. He had some volunteers staying who were offering their services in any humanitarian field. This sounded too good to be true so I went over to meet them and found these nine young men and women to be the answer to my prayers. They were such a great team comprising three couples and three individuals, all with different backgrounds and expertise. They were young, full of energy and – best of all – had a great sense of humour. Within a few days, we nicknamed them 'The Magnificent Nine'.

When Hope Worldwide didn't renew its funding for my band of merry helpers, incredibly seven of them stayed on for another six months to help me even though I had no money to pay them. As I told them, 'The river is flowing in the wrong direction for any of us to have a salary.' One of my lovely Magnificent Nine who became my personal assistant earned the nickname Jenny the General. She was such a great organizer that I miss her to this day, even though we are still in touch from afar. Another volunteer named Kara who helped with recordkeeping and administration was so moved when she watched me deliver a baby that when she returned to the States she enrolled in medical school and is now a doctor. I am indebted to all nine of them, and they will for ever remain part of our hospital family because – quite frankly – I would never have been able to finish my hospital on my own if they hadn't come to me when they did.

★★★

The Edna Adan Ismail Maternity Hospital took a lifetime to be born but that finally happened in March 2002, when it was officially opened and registered as a charity in perpetuity. I so often wondered if this day would ever come, but the gleaming white three-storey building bearing my father's name looked exactly like the one I'd dreamed of when I was a child. It not only stood as a testament against all those who thought it would never happen, but it rose from a site of death and misery to become a place were new lives would be brought into the world.

Even though we were open for business, there was still much to do with countless delays, obstructed shipments, unexpected cost overruns and periodic shortages of skilled labour that dragged the construction work on and on. We had originally planned the opening for International Women's Day on 8 March, an appropriate day to launch a maternity hospital. But by then the UN and our own government had scheduled so many other functions to mark the day that there would have been no officials free so we settled on 9 March instead.

I was delighted and proud that President Mohamed Egal agreed to inaugurate our building and we lined up a video crew specially to film the occasion. There was so much to do ahead of the big day, including deciding where to place the podium, how to arrange the guest seating and rope off the expected crowds, and where to site the security checkpoints to screen visitors. Mohamed happened to be my first husband and a dear friend, but he was also our head of state so his security guards had to survey the grounds and stake out the streets and buildings around the hospital compound to prevent any potential troublemakers from attempting to disrupt the proceedings, or maybe attempt to assassinate him.

As we scrambled to make the necessary preparations, I remember thinking how much I now appreciated the advanced planning that must have gone into all those diplomatic trips Mohamed and I took during his years as Prime Minister. I remembered being surprised by the numbers of armed secret service agents at the White House, but now I was the one worrying about receiving a President. I worked for weeks in advance to ensure that the occasion would come off safely for everybody. And then something totally unexpected happened; something which none of us could have prepared for. At 8 a.m. on the morning of the opening, Mohamed rang me to say he could not make it to the ceremony. I was stunned and angry and my immediate thought was that he was just being lazy.

'No, Mohamed! Come on, don't tell me this now!' I berated. 'You promised! I am sure you can make it. Just come and open my hospital, then you can leave.'

He sounded extremely weary when he said, 'I can't, Edna. I am calling you from my sickbed. I am really not well. I am so sorry to miss this, but I promise that I will come and see it another time. I simply cannot get out of bed today. I will send the Vice President instead.'

'But you can't do this to me, Mohamed! This is the biggest day of my life. Maybe I could postpone the opening until you're better?' I heard myself say, even though we both knew that wasn't possible.

'Believe me, there is nowhere I would like to be more than at your side today, Edna, but I just can't. I'm sorry.'

I was so upset as I was genuinely looking forward to having him there to cut the ribbon on this momentous day. Edna Hospital would not exist if it weren't for Mohamed. He had known me in London as a student nurse. He remembered my father and what he'd meant to me. Mohamed, of all people, knew how important this was to me and how it had been my burning ambition since

I was twelve years old. I don't think he ever really understood what drove me to do it but once he saw my determination to proceed, he gave me his blessing, the official permission and the land to build it on. Whenever he arrived back in Somaliland from a foreign visit, he would even instruct his driver to drive past the hospital to see its progress as he felt so emotionally invested in it.

Tempted as I was to cancel the opening and wait until he was better, I knew the event had to go on. I choked back my disappointment but his absence ruined my day. Devastated, I scrambled to change my opening speech, which began with, 'Welcome, Mr. President', and was full of anecdotes such as: 'I remember the first time President Egal suggested this place to me as the potential site for my hospital, and the day I sat here on this former garbage dump and tried to imagine what the future hospital might look like.' None of these memories would mean anything to the Vice President of the Republic of Somaliland, Dahir Riyale Kahin, whom I hardly knew.

To his credit, Riyale did a fine job. He opened the hospital and led the procession inside to tour the operating theatre, and maternity and paediatric wards. Some of the rooms were still unfinished, but that meant nothing to the mothers who had waited for so long. Though Mohamed couldn't be there in person, as I had hoped, the opening of the Edna Hospital undoubtedly reflected his spirit of optimism. There were drummers and dancers, speeches by politicians, health professionals, and members of the hospital board who had been so supportive during the construction. Following the formalities, the guests – including a swathe of dignitaries including the wife of the Italian ambassador for Somalia and those representing the UNHCR, WHO and UNICEF, along with several other international organizations – enjoyed a banquet of sambusas, meats and sweets. Whenever I look at the video footage of that day, it reminds me how far my dream had come.

When everyone had left and the dignitaries had driven off in a cloud of dust along with all the townspeople who'd come to have a good look at *their* hospital, I walked around the empty wards and rooms on my own and imagined what Dad would have thought of it all if he had lived long enough to see it. I think he would have been amazed and said something like, 'Wow! You did this, Shukri? That's my girl!' Or at least I hope that is what he would say.

Life often has a way of giving us deep sorrow and great joy in quick succession. Once all the fuss was over my staff and I still had work to do. We rolled up our sleeves, cleaned up the compound and re-scrubbed all the hospital floors and walls in preparation for our first patients. We worked until midnight until finally, exhausted, I climbed the stairs to my room and took a shower with the little remaining energy I had after a day crammed with emotions. I fell gratefully into my bed, and planned to open the doors to the public at 8 a.m. the following day. But at four in the morning someone started banging at the gate in the dark. A woman in labour had been brought in by her relatives – our first maternity patient. Four hours later we celebrated the birth of her child – our first delivery – at 8 a.m. on the morning of 10 March 2002. His name was Harir and I was photographed in my green scrubs and hairnet proudly holding him up to the camera. The son of a local policeman, Harir is a big guy now and knows us as if we are family. As our 'first-born', we offered him five years' free childcare, so he came to us for all his check-ups and vaccinations as we recorded his weight and height, checked his vital signs and fixed anything that wasn't right. Harir's little sister was born at the hospital a couple of years later. I caught up with them both recently and Harir informed me that he planned to be a doctor and work in our hospital one day. I was so thrilled at the prospect that I promised to contribute to his medical education if he performed well enough in secondary school.

In the months following the opening of the hospital, other women came to check us out and to see if we could deliver their babies. Before too long word got out that we could. In fact, since the day we first opened our doors our hospital has averaged between one and two hundred births a month. The original plan was always that it would be a non-profit maternity hospital with wards and outpatients for pre-natal and post-natal care, plus paediatrics. I added gynaecology because I wanted a fertility clinic that could help women have the babies that I could not. I remember how much I'd longed for a child and wanted to provide for those who felt the same way.

My plans for the hospital's remit changed less than twenty-four hours after we'd opened when an eighty-year-old man was knocked down in the street by a donkey cart right opposite our entrance. Once he fell he cracked his head and was bleeding heavily, so people carried him in like a sack of potatoes, holding his arms and legs as he dripped blood all over my clean floor. One of my security staff objected to them bringing him to us, reminding the crowd that we were a small maternity hospital that dealt only with pregnant women. Overruling him, I said, 'Let him in. Don't waste time talking about it. Let's just stop the bleeding and then you can worry about whether he is pregnant or not!' We did that and then we stitched him up. Because he was concussed and didn't know who he was or where he came from, we kept him in overnight – our first male patient. His relatives came and found him the next day, by which time he was conscious and talking. A few days later, he returned to have his stitches removed, so we had inadvertently become a general hospital.

From that day on, I knew that we couldn't turn anyone away. People would only ask, 'Why him and why not us?' And they came in their droves – with everything from a severe asthma attack to a diabetic coma. How could I say no? Before too long, I opened a male ward for patients with every condition – scorpion bites, burns, landmine victims, cleft palates, snake bites, accidental poisonings, kids drinking kerosene, malaria, hepatitis, meningitis, shingles, measles, the lot. We are now a leading hospital for the treatment of everything from hydrocephalus to fistulas, AIDS to road accidents, and we treat patients of all ages and both genders, regardless of their ability to pay. We are also the place where premature babies are cared for, regardless of where they were born. The hospital now has a diagnostic laboratory, an emergency blood bank, and provides treatment for sexually transmitted diseases. Facilities are available for medical research, studies and counselling, and we are fighting everything from infant mortality to AIDS. We have been helped and supported by so many kind people and wonderful organizations, such as the ninety-four-year-old Australian gynaecologist Dr Catherine Hamlin and her Fistula Hospital in Addis Ababa who sent me her deputy for a month and who repaired forty-five women for us. Later, the Fistula Foundation came onboard and generously covers the costs of all fistula surgery for any woman in my care.

My friends often say that my hospital is like a husband to me. If so, it would be my fourth. I have already lived with this one longer than I ever did with my previous three, even though it has demanded far more from me than any of the others. I suspect I had been looking for this husband from the time I was a girl called Shukri, growing up in my father's shadow. God willing, I will stay with this one until my last breath.

Best of all, I know that Dad would have been proud of me, because he never failed to tell me so when he was alive. I felt that he was with us on the day my hospital opened and I am sure has been with me ever since. I think about him often, even today, especially when I feel too exhausted to do something that needs to be done; at those moments, the recollection of my father's dedication pushes me to keep going. I hope it is the hospital he would have wanted. It does have its limitations but I have executed it to the best of my ability and it has grown beyond all my expectations. One thing is for sure – my father is with me in spirit every time we deliver another baby. Looking to the sky whenever a new life comes into this world, I secretly ask, 'I hope you're seeing this, Dad? I hope I did the right thing?' I think I know what he would say.

Epilogue

I was having lunch with the Italian ambassador to Somalia in Nairobi, Kenya in May 2002 when his wife informed me of a report that Mohamed Egal had died. She assured me that it looked to be a false alarm as he had gone onto the radio to tell everyone that he was okay.

I knew his health had deteriorated recently and that he'd been flown to Pretoria in South Africa for treatment, but I hadn't seen him since he'd been unable to attend the hospital opening two months earlier, so I knew nothing more. Worried for him throughout the lunch and later at the conference on maternal child health that I was in Kenya for, I returned to my hotel room and considered calling his wife to see how he was. Before I could, the telephone rang. It was the Italian ambassador's wife. 'Edna dear, I am sorry to tell you that Mohamed Egal is dead. He had a second cardiac arrest and passed away in hospital. He was having surgery for cancer and his bowel perforated.'

My legs gave way beneath me and I sat down hard on my bed. Mohamed seemed indestructible; he had survived so much. He was the only man I had ever truly loved and the news cut me to the quick. I wept as hard for him then as I did for my father. I wept for Somaliland and I wept for my people.

His body was flown home from South Africa and he received

a state funeral that – just as with my father – I couldn't attend. If I had been in the country, I would have fought for the right to be there. I visited his grave in Berbera later, but in the same way as Dad's bleak tombstone in Mogadishu had no meaning for me, neither did Mohamed's. When I finally accepted that he really was gone and that I would never be able to seek his counsel again, I couldn't help but reflect back to when we'd first met at a ball in London almost fifty years earlier. With his flashy red sports car and his rather arrogant proposal later via my father, he was a young man full of confidence and hope for the future.

We had lived through so much together with imprisonment, persecution, near bankruptcy, multiple losses and a devastating civil war. The chief thing we had in common was our love for Somaliland and our determination not to give up on her. Time and again, he especially had risked everything to fight for our people and their right to live in safety and good health. He was single-handedly responsible for saving us from the clutches of Somalia and helping us break away. The son of the richest man in Somaliland, he lost everything he owned thanks to Siad Barre, and when his first wife grew old and sick, it was I who cared for her in hospital and paid her bills.

To this day I believe that Mohamed was the best thing that ever happened to my country. There must be some higher power that decided that things had gone so badly for our people that there was an urgent need for a strong and savvy leader, someone to sort things out and set us on a new track. I cannot think of anyone else who could have played that role so well. From 1993 when he was elected President of a nation that was totally destroyed, only somebody like Mohamed could have pulled it back and fixed things in nine short years. He helped develop the Constitution and established a Parliament with a House of Representatives and a House of Elders. He worked for reconciliation among the clans, pressed for the voluntary demobilization of the rival militias, and established democratically elected political parties. Under his leadership, Somaliland introduced its own currency, passports and postage stamps, and began to collect taxes from businessmen and livestock exporters. He laid down the foundation that enabled Somaliland to make the progress it did, in spite of a shocking lack of formal recognition by the international community. Even when Britain and the rest of the world turned its back on us and refused to accept our national democratic vote to separate from Somalia – a situation that still exists today – Mohamed refused to be bowed.

The foundations he laid have even been strong enough to survive the inefficiencies and incompetence of later governments. People often talk about Somaliland as a 'rare African miracle'. I couldn't agree more, but that 'miracle' required human agency and strong leadership at a critical moment in our country's history. Mohamed was someone whom I will always love, respect and admire. He had a passion for his people and his country. Somaliland is where it is today because of him.

★★★

It was in part because of Mohamed that three months after his death I bowed to pressure and accepted the role of Minister of Family Welfare and Social Development, becoming Somaliland's first ever female minister with portfolio.

This was a brand new ministry designed to garner female votes and had been created by the government without much thought as to how it would be run and what it would do. I ended up feeling as if I was merely a quota, the woman in the cabinet and a symbolic

presence; someone who'd been appointed at a time when I was
so busy that they probably thought I wouldn't have time to be
much of a nuisance. When I arrived at my first cabinet meeting
they didn't even have a chair for me. There wasn't even a ministry
for me to work from so I set myself up on the empty top floor of
the hospital and ran it from there, telling people, 'When I'm on
the ground floor I'm a midwife. When I'm on the first floor I am
Edna, and when I'm upstairs I am the Minister.'

I negotiated that I would only be the Minister for fifty per cent
of the time as I was still 'breastfeeding' my baby – my hospital –
which continued to demand so much of my time and attention.
I remained in my generally ineffective cabinet position until the
next elections eight months later when I was elected the Minister
for Foreign Affairs, a job I had truly been born to do. This at least
had a clear purpose, as my role was to meet with governments,
open talks and diplomatic offices, appoint people and plan for the
future. In other words, the kind of public relations work I'd been
doing all my life. I travelled all over the world and often many
times to the same countries, especially in the European Union,
USA, UK and Scandinavia. It was my personal mission and my
dearest wish to persuade the world that our country had been the
British Somaliland Protectorate, which gained its independence
from Britain in 1960 when neighbouring Italian Somalia was still
under colonial rule. Somaliland therefore was not a breakaway
region of Somalia but a country older than Italian Somalia, with
legitimate and internationally defined boundaries that should be
formally recognized as an independent sovereign state. We want
our own legitimate identity, a place at the table and a voice on
international platforms. Currently we are not represented at the
UN, the Arab League or the African Union – only Somalia is.
Quite unjustly, we don't even appear on any map!

First of all, though, I understood that it was important to let the world know exactly who, what and where we were. All they'd ever heard about us from Somalia was that the people of Somaliland were dissidents and rebels who had wilfully disrupted their country and challenged their territorial integrity, when the opposite was the truth. By being ignored for so long we were being punished for the crimes of Somalia, which was being rewarded with billions of dollars worth of foreign taxpayers' money and by the presence of thousands of international peacekeeping forces. I pleaded with the African Union to come on a fact-finding mission to Somaliland and see how peaceful, democratic and stable we were in comparison to the chaos created by the Mogadishu warlords. A delegation eventually arrived in 2005 and wrote an extremely positive report, which felt to us like a huge victory, until we realized that hardly anybody read it and no one was prepared to be the first to act on it. They were not only fearful of repercussions from Somalia but the accusation that their support could lead to the disintegration of the African Union. They argued, and still argue, that it is only for Somalia to agree to our separation, when Somalia has no legal ownership over Somaliland. In short, the world has allowed Somalia, the aggressor, to represent Somaliland, the victim – which is a bit like appointing Adolf Hitler to defend the rights of those he put into concentration camps.

I have repeatedly argued that all we are trying to do in Somaliland is go back to the way we were before our disastrous union. This is exactly what Senegal and Gambia did when their brief unification didn't work out, and the same with Egypt and Syria. None of those countries were punished for voluntarily uniting with another country before democratically changing their minds and separating again. Somehow, Somaliland has remained voiceless and invisible to the world for over twenty-eight years. My people feel very let down by our former allies like the European Union and America, and especially betrayed by the British – whom we felt should have supported their former protectorate. Instead, as a breakaway country that doesn't officially exist we have to fight for every scrap or morsel from the vast international developmental aid that is sent to Somalia and which largely bypasses us. All we qualify for is a trickle of humanitarian aid. Even when it comes to fundraising for my hospital, I have to make it crystal clear that we have nothing to do with terrorists and pirates and that any money donated will go directly to purchase bedpans and syringes and not into the pockets of warlords to buy them bombs and bazookas.

As Foreign Minister, I knew that change wouldn't happen overnight, but I hoped to get people to at least accept that our desire for a divorce from Somalia was not only legal, but also justified in light of our history. Frustratingly, it was one of the few missions I failed in and one in which every one of my successors has come up against the same obstacles. To this day, the people of Somaliland have been denied a hearing and their day in court.

I remained in the cabinet for three years but my hospital suffered without me working there every day and my own health suffered too. In 2005 I almost died of pneumonia and pleurisy and was also concerned about the precarious finances of my facility that was now deeply in the red. I had done everything I could do as a diplomat and in 2006 I felt that it was time to step out. Politics might not have been quite done with me – I'm still called upon for advice and consultation, to speak to delegations as a special envoy, and sent on missions – but I was done with it. One thing I am proud of, though, is the fact that I am almost certainly the only foreign minister in the world to have delivered triplets while still in office.

★★★

The year after the Edna Hospital opened and some time after
Mohamed's passing, my mother Marian died. She was ninety-two
and lived in London with my sister Asha and had become my
financial dependent. Relatives cared for her in west London but
I paid for her accommodation and all her needs until the end.
Farah and Asha and I arranged for her funeral in Hertfordshire,
UK, not far from Clare Hospital where my father and I had both
worked.

Because of her dementia, Mum never really knew what I'd
achieved. In the early days whenever I told her of my plans, she'd
ask me, 'But why are you building a hospital?'

'Because I want to.'

'But you're not a builder, Edna. Why doesn't the government
build it?'

'The government is building its own hospitals. I want to build
my own so that I can treat women the way I think they should
be treated. I want to train nurses the way I think they should be
trained. I want things done my way, and I need to be in charge.'

'But why you?'

Towards the end of her life, she became a frail old lady and one
with whom I made my peace. Sweetly, even when she couldn't
recall much else, she could still remember the words of the songs
she used to sing to on her old gramophone, playing the records
my father used to bring her back from his trips. She'd always had
a lovely singing voice and one of my most precious possessions
is a tape recording of Mum singing when she was ninety-one, a
year before she died. It is a shame that my mother never really
understood how much satisfaction and pleasure my work gave
me, or realized just how blessed I have been. I could have been

a millionaire twice over with my history and connections but as I've never taken a salary from the hospital and have used up all my savings, I will probably die as poor as my father was. Yet I am the richest woman in the world. I measure my wealth not in money or camels but in the lives I have brought into this world and those I have saved. Building the hospital was my way of healing after so much heartbreak. Keeping it running is my choice. Why do people climb Mount Everest? It's because they have to. The hospital is my Mount Everest.

The woman who gave me the name Edna is buried in a cemetery in Hertfordshire, UK, eight thousand kilometres from Somaliland. If ever I wanted to move my father's remains from Somalia to lie alongside her then that was made impossible when the huge Mogadishu cemetery where he was interred was bulldozed to make way for housing. I will never go back there. When I was growing up, I was almost certainly the only Edna in the country. Now there are hundreds of Ednas as Somalilanders often choose to give their daughters my name. We have at least two Ednas working in my hospital including an anaesthetist known as 'Little Edna', the eldest of eleven, who was so small and frail when she came to me as a teenager that I was initially reluctant to admit her. What tipped the balance for me was the fact that, once she was trained, she would be the only breadwinner for her family. She proved to be a superb midwife and anaesthetist and is now a trainer of anaesthetists. When Little Edna is on duty, I can sleep well. She would make a great candidate for medical school.

Almost everyone I talk to tells me that they hope their daughters will become nurses one day and work with me. 'We want her to be just like you,' they say.

'No,' I correct them, 'not like me. Better.'

When I advertised for my first forty nurses once my hospital was complete, well over three hundred applied. This reversal from my earliest recruiting efforts when nursing was considered beneath the dignity of most is flattering and humbling. Our profession is now not only regarded as respectable for girls, but also highly desirable. Delivering babies and helping women is empowering to the young midwives and nurses and a source of pride for their parents, who lobby me relentlessly to approve their daughters' admission to our programme.

Every day, when I go to work and teach these young girls how to be the best they can be, I am inspired not only by my father but by all the remarkable health professionals who made such an impression on me. When I opened my operating theatres and had to train my nurses I invoked the memory of Tiger Monk, making them learn the hard way, doing dry run after dry run with dummies in the lab or instruments in the sterilizing room before they went near any live surgery. I am also ever mindful of the tragedies that affected my parents, with the loss of a baby sister to a forceps birth and the death of my brother from being dropped. These memories help motivate my mission to prevent other families suffering what we did. Anyone who knows me will tell you that I have fits if I see my students being careless with the precious young lives they hold in their arms.

★★★

Dad is never far from my thoughts but especially when I teach midwives in the hospitals in Berbera or Erigavo – two places that bring back a flood of emotions. Even the smell of the ocean in Berbera takes me back. In those hospitals especially I climb the steps my father climbed and walk the floors he walked. I try to remember his lessons in confidence building when my own nursing students are struggling to stick to their studies, and am freshly inspired by those who go on to surprise and delight me. I may not have had children of my own but I have all the babies that I've brought into the world, and these young girls whose lives I have changed. I remember many of them as timid student nurses, frightened of everything, and then I watched them grow in confidence and go on to become the doctor that I would have liked to be. Yesterday they were my students. Then they became my colleagues. Now they are my superiors. More than half of my clinical residents are women. This is my evolution.

My hospital's Associate Director Shukri Mohamed Dahir is just such an example, and not just because her name is Shukri. When she first came to me eighteen years ago I didn't expect her to last a week. She and her family had fled the 1988 bombings in Hargeisa, so she grew up in a refugee camp. She received her basic education in what were called 'Nido Schools' after the empty powdered milk tins that served as seats for the pupils. She lied about her age to get into our programme, claiming she was eighteen when she was really fifteen, but once she started there was no doubt that she would be a star. Her performance quickly earned my confidence and I helped finance her through medical school. She is now as invaluable to me as my right hand. Shukri had the grit and our training gave her the confidence to become a successful nurse, midwife, doctor, surgeon and health educator. The irony is that even though we have come so far, I still have male patients and relatives who insist on any surgery being performed by a man, and especially by a white doctor. Whenever that happens I ask one of our drivers or a European to step in and pretend to be a doctor just to keep them happy. Then, once the patients are under anaesthetic, Shukri or any one of her talented female counterparts take over.

In reality, women have come a long way in Somaliland. Even though we also have male doctors and nurses, the stars somehow aligned and we now have a female senior surgeon, a female assistant surgeon, a female instrument nurse, a female anaesthetist, a female theatre supervisor, all operating on a male patient in a hospital owned by a female. To me, this is living proof of our progress

Then there is the trainer of my midwives, Ridwan Mohamoud, whose father was assigned to me as a bodyguard when I was Foreign Minister. He was forever telling me how clever his daughter was, so I sent her books, paper and pens to encourage her to read and write. Her father suffered a stroke and then died a few years later, leaving a wife and sixteen children. With my help Ridwan graduated among the top students in my midwifery school and now works for me as a Clinical Instructor. Her youngest sister is also in training, so the family will soon have two incomes. This is what I live for, as well as all those we've helped through what I call my 'ten-dollar collections' – in which I asked for ten dollars apiece from friends and colleagues to pay for anything from a small stipend for widows, or funds to give an orphan an education. Whenever I walk down the street in Hargeisa, I can't move for people calling out, 'Edna! Edna!' or *'Edo! Edo!'* (Auntie), eager to tell me that they were born in my hospital, that their sister or their aunt or their mother was trained by me, or that my father saved the life of their grandmother.

★★★

My hospital runs on the kindness, professionalism and encouragement of my staff, my friends and neighbours, my former colleagues, volunteers, governmental and non-governmental organizations, and our many donors and supporters worldwide. We still don't have our own well, so all our water has to be transported in from forty-five kilometres away at huge expense. There is no oxygen readily available in Somaliland so we make our own with oxygen concentrator machines that require electricity, which in turn require fuel. All of our equipment is imported and much of it secondhand. Just like the incubator donated to the Medina Hospital from a grateful patient, we now have an old ambulance from the UN Refugee Agency, a generator from the Danish Refugee Council, a water tanker from a Somali businessman, an ultrasound machine from a visiting German doctor who sent us his old one, two incubators from the Dutch, a wheelchair from Greece, and a refrigerator for blood from a Somali who owed me a favour. My first computer came from a Somali in London who was about to throw it away for a new one, and the mobile pulse oxygen oxymeters my senior staff use are mostly donated too. My outpatients department and a laboratory were built with a grant from USAID and the British gave us beds, baby cots and equipped our operating theatre – all of which are all still being used after eighteen years.

With much more to achieve and more support to seek I have a million reasons to get up each morning and work for an average ten hours every day, despite my eight decades on this earth. There is still so much to do, from challenging the Somali superstition that branding a baby's chest will prevent TB to driving hundreds of miles in convoys to distribute fortified lentils to mother and child centres, schools and drought-affected communities, where we try to educate people about healthy eating – 'You feed spinach to your goats but you need to eat it too.' Every week the numbers of patients brought in to us from the bush threatens to overwhelm us. We still have mothers dying of complications such as toxaemia and eclampsia that no longer kill women in the West but are the biggest killers in Somaliland, where seventy per cent of the people live not in cities but in poor nomadic communities without any healthcare. We have women brought in after a gruelling five-day journey while in labour or with the placenta still inside them one week after their baby was born. One mother arrived with her dead baby still inside her, minus its arm, which was pulled off by her traumatized nine-year-old daughter enlisted to assist her when the baby was lying across the pelvis and an arm prolapsed. Some of these patients die on our doorstep. Others die soon after admission. Most of the mothers and babies could have been saved if they'd had basic pre-natal care or had come to us sooner, or if those attending to them had some knowledge of midwifery or medical care. Knowledge is the most valuable gift we can give to our people and pass on to future generations.

To date and with the help of my trained staff we have delivered over 25,000 babies, many of whom would have otherwise died. Since 2011 my hospital has been the Edna Adan University Hospital in which we train doctors, pharmacists, laboratory technicians and health educators as well as nurses and midwives for the entire region. We also offer a post-graduate mother and child health diploma courses for doctors and a Bachelor of Science degree in all aspects of nursing, midwifery and public health. Over a thousand midwives, and hundreds of nurses, anaesthetists, pharmacists and lab technicians have gone back to their villages or out into the world with their qualifications from my hospital or from one of our seven training schools across the country. In their colour-coded uniforms – red for community midwives, green for the pharmacists, blue for the nursing students and so on, they go where they are most needed. The skilled medical work they do and the training they provide not only brings about significant changes in those communities but encourages others to seek an education also.

The fees we charge are a fraction of Western costs and are very often paid for by various charitable organizations and our many support groups around the world, some of whom came to know of me from further articles written about me in the *New York Times* and a chapter about me in the book *Half the Sky: How to Change the World* by Pulitzer prize-winning journalists Nicholas Kristof and Sheryl WuDunn, published in 2009. I also became known for my TED talks and for the many international awards I began to receive, such as the French *Légion d'honneur,* honorary PhDs from Clark University in Massachusetts, Ahfad University for Women in the Sudan, the University of Pennsylvania, London South Bank and Cardiff University. Also much appreciated is the Chancellor's Medal for my 'outstanding contribution to Human Rights' awarded by the University of Pretoria.

I have also never stopped campaigning against FGM, still too prevalent in my part of the world with an estimated three million girls cut annually in Africa alone. As part of our determined fight against female circumcision, in 2018 we were able to win the support of the *mufti*, Somaliland's top religious authority to pronounce a *fatwa* that condemns Type 3 FGM. This is the first of its kind in Africa and will hopefully encourage many more countries to follow suit. We secured the same kind of condemnation from the WHO, which has declared FGM a violation of human rights. In spite of such damning declarations, this hidden practice still goes on. Just recently we saved the life of an eleven-year-old girl with Down's Syndrome who fought so violently against the woman circumcising her that she almost died from a loss of blood. By the time her family finally brought her in to us, she needed a couple of units of blood. Her urethra and everything else had been cut to the bone and she now faces a life of incontinence and other problems. It was the worst thing I have ever seen in my long nursing career and, although we saved her life, she will never be free of the consequences or the trauma. Although illegal, FGM is also still practised elsewhere in the world and, through migration, British, European, US and other midwives are having to deal with the consequences. In February 2019, a Ugandan mother became the first woman to be found guilty of FGM in the UK. Her three-year-old daughter had to be taken to hospital with severe bleeding after being held down and cut. She had lost a significant amount of blood and doctors alerted the police. It was only the fourth FGM prosecution in the UK and the first three ended in acquittals. In the US, similar cases have also collapsed and a Detroit judge recently ruled that the 1996 law passed by Congress banning the practice nationwide was 'unconstitutional' and should be outlawed by individual states. His ruling led to the dismissal of all charges against a female doctor who cut nine girls aged between six and eight. The fight to prevent this barbaric practice from happening is far from over.

Also not over is my campaign to improve healthcare in our country. The nursing and medical students whose training I have paid for and sweated over have collectively contributed towards the overall peace, stability and economic growth that our people have enjoyed for the past twenty-eight years. With their help, since the end of the civil war our infant mortality rate – which was one of the world's highest – has fallen to a quarter of its pre-war high. Maternal mortality has fallen too, from 1,600 to around 300 per 100,000 births, compared to around twelve per 100,000 in developed countries. Sadly, we have still lost sixty-seven mothers – the majority to eclampsia because they never attended pre-natal clinics to have their blood pressure taken or their health monitored. Those are sixty-seven mothers too many and I am doing all I can to reduce that number to zero. It will be my legacy.

Sadly, the students I need to achieve this and so much more are being systematically poached from abroad by hospitals and international organizations. These are often the same people who tell us they don't have the funds to help us with training and offer us nothing towards our costs, but then send scouts to lure away my best doctors, nurses and midwives the moment they qualify. I now have former students working in America, Canada, Norway, Europe and all over the world, a brain drain that makes us proud and helps us measure ourselves against other institutions. But it can also make me feel as though these wealthy people are breaking into my home, opening my safe and stealing my time, my energy and my resources. What they are doing lays to waste some of my life's work and is a form of human piracy I can do nothing about.

★★★

People are always asking me when I might retire, but why slow down if the engine is still running? One of my favourite songs is Edith Piaf's 'No Regrets' but aside from wishing I'd punched a few more noses, I do have one regret – that I turned down the opportunity to study medicine when it was offered to me in London.

In my dotage, I have even considered going back to school myself because I think not becoming a doctor may have been the biggest mistake of my life. Sometimes at two o'clock in the morning when I have a woman bleeding and I have to send the ambulance to fetch a doctor who doesn't really want to come out at that hour, I think, 'If only I'd done medicine, I could have done this C-section myself.' The doctors who work for me or help me out have been incredible. Quite recently a baby was born on my labour ward with its large intestines delivered afterwards like a snake. Without immediate surgery he would die. Our doctors had never operated on anything like this before so I immediately thought of Dr Suleiman, the best surgeon in Somaliland and twice Minister of Health, who now runs a private hospital. In 1994 when I was with the WHO, I sent him to Switzerland for training, so he owes me – a fact I remind him of frequently. I called him, explained the situation and said, 'I need you right away.'

'I'll be there in twenty minutes,' he replied. 'Have the operating theatre ready.' By the time he arrived, Dr Shukri had my intensive care team fully prepared with anaesthetists and assistant surgeons scrubbed up. The long and complicated operation was successful and the baby went home with its happy mother a few weeks later. And of course it was all free of charge, because the woman came from the bush. I can't put a price on that kind of care and that's exactly the kind of patient I built this hospital for. My staff and I are proud and honoured to have saved that child. He's certainly a fighter and could become a President of the Republic one day, who knows? Or better still a doctor in my hospital.

I still imagine that if I were ten years younger I would retrain as a surgeon but in many ways, I am glad that I didn't. I don't think I could have spent the rest of my life locked up in operating theatres. I'd have missed all the babies and the decision-making in midwifery, which is equally fast. The authority and responsibility you carry is enormous to make sure that mother and baby survive. If I'd been swallowed up into the world of physicians, healthcare would have remained in the hands of doctors in Somaliland, nurses wouldn't have achieved their current status, girls might not have taken up the profession, and fewer women would have had jobs. Midwifery especially would never have developed as it has and I doubt that Somaliland would have achieved the status of having the biggest per capita number of trained midwives in Africa. If we could set a goal of training one million midwives on our continent over the next decade, I can die knowing that the experience of childbirth and the needless suffering of Africa's women will forever be changed.

Despite the many challenges, frustrations and setbacks I have faced – and continue to face on a daily basis – it is my belief in the future health of my country which keeps me working even harder than ever. I know that I won't always be able to keep going at this pace or keep making the kinds of sacrifices I have made and because of this I have finally learned to delegate – the one thing my father would have advised me to do a long time ago. I have spent all my money and only have my UN pension to live on and to pay for the things I need for the hospital, and when I die that pension will die too. Some people think that I own the hospital but, in truth, it owns me. I have set up a legal trust so that it can never be sold and will always be a place for the provision of subsidised or free healthcare. I hope to find someone as passionate as my father to take it over; someone who has the same sense of courage and commitment, duty, ethics and determination, someone who will protect my hospital, swim with it and defend it.

In 2017, at the age of eighty, I was invited to serve in the independent Council of Elders to oversee future Somaliland elections. My fellow committee members include three former Vice Presidents. I want my people to aim for excellence, to compete with themselves and get better each time. We come from a poor, developing country but I don't want them to think that means we come from a disadvantaged background. I tell them, 'Don't say you

316   EDNA ADAN ISMAIL

have nothing. You have a brain and that is everything. You should give up saying "I cannot do" and say instead "I will try to do".'

Teacher training is another big focus of mine to maintain the quality of education in our country and create a trickle-down effect. My mantra has always been, 'If I don't do it then who will?' and this is yet another example. Ever since I was denied the opportunity to learn as a little girl, things have changed dramatically in Somaliland, but there are still so many young people who do not have access to the same opportunities that were offered to me. One of the worst legacies Siad Barre left us with was that an entire generation grew up in refugee camps where they learned how to read and write by making marks in the sand. Sadly, they also learned that the smart people are those who make easy money, look for shortcuts and get away with things. This is in danger of becoming a national mentality. I will do all I can to make sure that they not only learn how to read, write and do their sums, but also learn respect, dignity and pride in our country. I want them to know that it is wrong to lie, to steal or to cheat, to spit or break things. If they don't learn this from the parents then it has to come from the teachers who need to be taught how to fully engage and encourage their pupils, as they did with me.

In 2018, I was delighted to be awarded an honorary doctorate at the London South Bank University, the new name for the Borough Polytechnic where I'd attended my pre-nursing course in the 1950s. It was surprisingly emotional to put on the blue and black gown and cap and tell five hundred people how profoundly humbled and grateful this honour felt for 'a skinny seventeen-year-old girl on a scholarship from British Somaliland'. I added, 'The education and training that I received here prepared me for all the subsequent and varied responsibilities that followed in my life... Today, not only do I take pride in all that Britain has taught me but I am also reminded of all the young people in my country who do not have access to the same opportunities that were offered to me when I was their age. This is the reason that makes me devote as much energy as I can to make available to our youth the most precious gift that was ever given to me, which is the gift of education.' I concluded with thanks to my parents who, I said, 'saw my hunger for learning and who spared no effort to help me pursue my professional ambitions.'

In Hargeisa after the war, my father hired a tutor for the neighbourhood children because he wanted them to be better educated – and me too, by default. He instilled in me such a strong sense of honour, determination and discipline, for which I thank him every day. It isn't just my hospital that stands testament to him and all that he stood for: it is me, and all those I have sent out into the world in his name. In sha'Allah, their light will continue to shine long after I am buried in the red dirt of Somaliland, where my epitaph should probably be – 'She was crazy but she tried.' I am not ready to hang up my midwife's uniform just yet, though. I still have work to do and bills to pay and people to sponsor and nurses and doctors to send out into the world to practise what I have preached. It would kill me not to be needed or to have a challenge. I was born with the drive to fix things. I can't imagine not working and I hope to die with my proverbial boots on.

I recently appeared on the BBC's *Desert Island Discs* programme and had to nominate the eight records that meant the most to me. Aside from songs by Edith Piaf and Ella Fitzgerald, I chose a recording of the poet Robert Frost reading 'Stopping by Woods on a Snowy Evening', which I first heard at school in London. I chose it because it has such deep resonance for me, and especially the final line: 'For I have promises to keep, and miles to go before I sleep. And miles to go before I sleep...'

Give

Fifty per cent of all royalties received through the sale of this book will be donated by the family of Edna Adan Ismail to the Edna Adan University Hospital.

Please see charities below which support our work in Somaliland.

Edna Adan University Hospital, Somaliland

For more information about the Edna Adan University Hospital, visit http://www.ednahospitalfoundation.org

If you would like to support the work of the hospital, please visit the site of the Edna Adan Hospital Foundation at https://donatenow.networkforgood.org/EAHF

Friends of Edna

You may also donate directly to the Friends of Edna Endowment Fund to help ensure the sustainability of the hospital's training programmes, professional staff, and state-of-the-art physical plant for generations to come. Cheques to grow this endowment can be made out to 'Friends of Edna's Maternity Hospital' and sent to 95 Montgomery Street, Black Rock, CT 06605-3305, USA, for the attention of Dr Lee Cassanelli, President of Friends of the Edna Maternity Hospital while credit card donations should be directed through PayPal: donate@friendsofedna.org

Edna Adan Hospital Foundation
The Edna Adan Hospital Foundation is a 501 (c) (3) nonprofit organization (EIN 46-1552054) which supports the training of nurses and midwives, Female Genital Mutilation (FGM) community educational materials, necessary medical procedures, equipment and supplies, and has contributed to the construction of a new university building.

For more information, visit our website on https://ednahospital-foundation.org/#about

Support us by donating on https://donatenow.networkforgood.org/EAHF

If you prefer to contribute by check, please mail your check to: Edna Adan Hospital Foundation 1660 L Street NW Suite 501 Washington, DC 20036

Contact us on: Office: +1 (202) 849-0125Email: info@ednahospitalfoundation.org

Edna Foundation UK
We are an international non-profit organization working with the Edna Adan Hospital and University to advance health care in Somaliland and throughout the Horn of Africa. We promote safe motherhood by training midwives, fighting FGM and empowering women to step up as leaders of change.

Edna Adan Foundation Registered charity number 1169725

Fore more information visit us on www.ednafoundation.org.uk

Or contact us on contact@ednafoundation.org.uk

You can support us by donating here: https://www.justgiving. com/edna-adan-foundation

Whatever you donate, you will be helping to reduce maternal and infant mortality in the Horn of Africa by enabling safer pregnancies and deliveries. Thanks to Edna's free community midwifery training courses to students from distant villages and districts, you will be ensuring that newborn babies have access to immediate medical care, lifesaving vaccinations and, as they grow, quality health services.

You will be making certain that children's life chances are significantly increased so, when they're ready, they too can join the movement for improved healthcare in Somaliland by becoming trained health professionals. With your donations Edna and her team are able to train more midwives and expand their teaching programme to other areas of healthcare, including nursing, anaesthesiology, pharmacology, laboratory technology, dentistry, veterinary health, agriculture and public health. Your gifts also provide safe motherhood to women through clinics, supplies and, when necessary, C-section deliveries.

Whatever the circumstances, every baby born and every patient treated in Edna's hospital receives the best possible care they can provide. Your donation will not only make a difference but 100 per cent of any money gifted goes to this important work, especially to the poorest patients for whom all treatment is free, including delivery, C-sections, medication and hospital accommodation.

Acknowledgements

The list of the Edna Adan Hospital's supporters and partners is long and its well-wishers are many. In particular Edna would like to extend her thanks to her main supporters: the Friends of the Edna Maternity Hospital, the Edna Adan Hospital Foundation, and the Government of Somaliland, with special thanks to the Ministries of Health and Education. She also appreciates the partnership with SOFHA (Somaliland Family Health Association) with their work on FGM, sexual and reproductive health, and with numerous hospitals, universities and aid agencies around the world.

This story names most of those individuals who have helped Edna along her path. Many are no longer alive but her gratitude for them lives on and they are now recorded for posterity. She is also grateful for every single one of her students and staff and for all those who have given her encouragement, friendship and support, along with all the doctors, nurses and medical students from around the world who travel to Somaliland on a regular basis and volunteer to help in whatever their field of expertise.

Lee Cassanelli, author and Associate Professor of African History at the University of Pennsylvania, USA, sat with Edna over a period of five years and recorded thirty hours of taped interviews, which he transcribed and assembled into an invaluable chronological narrative of her recollections and reflections. British author Wendy Holden then spent an equivalent number of hours and used her own interview material and considerable writing skills to craft and perfect this book. Edna is indebted to them both.

Wendy and Edna are both grateful to Annabel Merullo at Peters Fraser Dunlop for all her hard work in facilitating this project and securing the film deal. Without her introduction and diligence, this book might never have happened. They would also like to thank Lisa Milton, Kate Fox and all the team at HQ for believing in it. Lastly, Wendy is thankful for Edna's love and friendship, and for the many inspirational lessons she has taught her about kindness, courage, determination and selflessness.

Edna Adan Ismail and Wendy Holden